Accident and Eme

A Structured Approac

Gary Jones SRN OND DN

Head of Accident and Emergency Nursing Services, Orsett and Basildon Hospitals, Essex; Chairman, RCN Accident & Emergency Nursing Association, UK

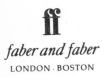

faber and faber

LONDON · BOSTON

First published in 1990
by Faber and Faber Limited
3 Queen Square London WC1N 3AU

Photoset by Parker Typesetting Service Leicester
Printed in England by Clays Ltd, St Ives plc

© Gary Jones, 1990

Gary Jones is hereby identified as author of this work in accordance with Section 77
of the Copyright, Designs and Patents Act 1988.

A CIP record for this book is available from the British Library

ISBN 0-571-14319-9

Contents

Foreword

If ever there was a time for a book to be written, this is the right time for this book. How many times have weread about the advances in accident and emergency nursing and nursing models, only to be discouraged by incomprehensible words and obtuse meanings. We have often felt that these do not apply – nor are they workable in an A & E department.

Gary Jones has turned away from these tomes, and from his own accident and emergency experience has written a sensible, easily read and much needed book. Of course, some nurses will say, we cannot do all this because of time or staff shortages. You should read this book, it can be studied in depth, in A & E departments, and in Colleges of Nursing, kept for reference and consulted during those rare moments of quiet in the department. Because of Gary Jones's hard work, planning and research in the preparation of this book, nurses will find their worries about the future of A & E nursing alleviated. Nurses who are looking for a nursing model or are planning changes in their departments will find their work made considerably easier by studying this book. Accident and emergency nursing has advanced rapidly in the past five years and is entering a further exciting phase. There is something for all nurses, from the learners to the most experienced A & E nurse in this book, and its greatest achievement is to take the misunderstood issues and make them understandable.

Kate O'Hanlon, MBE, RGN, RM
Cross of Merit,
Sovereign and Military Order of St John of Jerusalem Rhodes
and Malta
(Formerly Senior Sister, Accident & Emergency Department,
Royal Victoria Hospital, Belfast)

Preface and Acknowledgements

The use of nursing models, triage and a structured process of care in the Accident and Emergency department has been debated for many years. One of the main reasons for the apparent lack of progress is that many nurses have seen the introduction of such systems as merely an academic exercise, rather than providing a logical way of achieving a structured approach to the nursing care already in existence. This book aims to address these key issues and suggests a model of nursing, a triage system and process of care that can be used in any Accident and Emergency department.

Models are based on beliefs about humans who are the recipients of care. A model is simply a framework that provides a structure to care. If the suggested model of nursing is linked with a formalized triage system and then a problem-orientated approach is taken, a complete process of A & E nursing care can be achieved.

The 1990s provide the opportunity for us to develop our specialty. We can lift the service out of its Cinderella image and ensure Accident and Emergency nursing is identified in its true light – as a true specialty. The report 'A Strategy for Nursing' provides the targets at which all A & E nurses should be aiming; it allows for the development of primary nursing and the care of patients as individuals, with individual human needs.

In writing this book I was aware that any structure must be based on current nursing practice. To introduce a totally new approach to the care provided would merely alienate colleagues from my aim. The book has been produced in three sections. Part one comprises three chapters. The introduction introduces the reader to the subjects of nursing models, triage and the nursing process. It identifies the way forward and contains a philosophy for the A & E department. Chapter 2 introduces the reader to the Accident and Emergency Model of Nursing. The model is based on the belief that humans have seven components of life, comprising human behavioural, physical and social aspects. These components can be used in all stages of nursing care provided in the A & E setting. Chapter 3 provides a comprehensive guide to setting up a formalized triage system.

Part two of the book addresses the use of a formalized process of care. The chapters include patient assessment, analysing and planning care, intervention, evaluation and documentation. Throughout the chapters of this section, the model of nursing and triage system is used and integrated into the process.

The final section of the book uses a case history approach to identify how a structured approach to care can improve current practice and how the model can be used in nurse education. It ends with a self-evaluation chapter.

I am confident this book will help all Accident and Emergency nurses to structure their care and by so doing push back the boundaries of nursing and improve the already high standards that can be found in most A & E units in the UK.

So many people provided their thoughts and knowledge of accident and emergency nursing that identifying all the individuals by name would be impossible. I thank them all. Special thanks go to Kate O'Hanlon for providing the Foreword to this book. Her expertise and knowledge of trauma nursing, gained through the years at the Royal Victoria Hospital, Belfast, coupled with her compassion for patients as individuals, irrespective of their religious beliefs, provides a shining light for all humanity. To Lesley Green, Sister and Pat McKeogh, Staff Nurse at the Accident and Emergency Department, Orsett Hospital, my most sincere thanks. To all my staff many thanks for putting up with my constant pressure on them to develop and create new ways of improving and providing care. To June Hutson, my deepest and most sincere thanks for all the clerical work she has done and for typing this book. Finally to my parents, without whose support I would never have the time for such ventures as this book, or the work I undertake within the RCN Accident & Emergency Forum.

PART ONE

Developing the Process of Care in Accident and Emergency

1   *Introduction*

For as long as man has walked on the earth the great problem has been how to stay alive. There was, and to a certain extent still is, survival of the strongest and fittest. Despite this problem, development of a specialist service for victims of injury or sudden illness has been extremely slow. The publication by the Royal College of Surgeons on Trauma Care (1988) identified a major shortfall in the care of the severely traumatized patient.

The health and welfare of not only the individual but also the group became important as people began to live in communities. It became clear that everyone relied on each other to maintain the health and safety of the community and to assist each other when injured or unwell. This commitment to one's fellow human being was made more important with the emergence of christianity. In caring for the hurt and suffering you cared for God. This belief has had major implications for the development of nursing. God spoke to Florence Nightingale in 1837 and this led her into nursing and in 1854 to the battlefields of Scutari and her work during the Crimean War.

War has also had dramatic effects on the development of care for the injured, the most significant being the work of Jean Henri Dunant following his observations during the battle of Solferino. Dunant was the founder of the International Red Cross and the Convention of Geneva.

The development of accident and emergency services

Present-day accident and emergency departments have evolved from the casualty departments of the old voluntary hospitals and workhouses. Casualty departments provided care for all manner of problems. The major activity was primary, medical care for large sections of the population who could not obtain it from General Practitioners. In addition to this major activity the departments also catered for the injured.

With the advent of the National Health Service the primary role should have ceased, but even today a large percentage of attenders to accident and emergency departments are suffering from non-emergency conditions.

By 1959 it was clear to the then Minister of Health, that a major review was required into the casualty services. A report was published in 1962 (the Platt Report). The report made several key recommendations. Two of these were:

1 Casualty departments should change in function from providing primary care to casual attenders to the provision of a 24-hour accident and emergency service.
2 This service should be appropriately staffed, equipped and a named consultant should be identified.

The two major responsibilities of the accident and emergency service therefore had been identified:

1 The prime function was now to provide care for serious accident, medical and surgical emergencies.
2 The secondary or subsidiary function was to provide medical care for casual attenders.

Although these recommendations were accepted by the Minister and development of the specialty began, it was not until 1975 that the specialty of accident and emergency medicine officially came into being. It was named by an advisory committee, set up by the Royal Colleges of Physicians and Surgeons.

Accident and emergency nursing as a specialty

With the emergence of accident and emergency as a specialty in the late 1960s, it was a committed group of nurses who came together in 1972 to create the accident and emergency group within the

Royal College of Nursing. By 1978 this group had grown. It was very active in the development of accident and emergency nursing as a true nursing specialty, and was thus recognized as a major forum within the College. In 1975 the then Board of Clinical Nursing Studies created the Accident & Emergency Course, which today is still available through the National Boards. Accident and Emergency nurses therefore had, during the 1970s, placed accident and emergency nursing firmly on its feet and ensured its future progress.

This progress is still very evident today. Innovative developments such as the Nurse Practitioner, Triage Systems and Primary Nursing in Accident and Emergency, are all areas where accident and emergency nurses are pushing back the boundaries of nursing. A much slower development is the use of nursing models and the nursing process. This apparent shortcoming exists primarily because the development of models and the nursing process has been seen by many as an academic exercise, rather than a logical way of achieving a structured approach to the nursing care already in existence.

Steven Wright (1986) recognized that models are often seen as being unrealistic because they represent the views of a minority of academic nurses of what nursing ought to be. Millar said in 1985 that 'in trying to explain everything they explain nothing'.

Another major obstacle is the language barrier, which all too often conceals simple ideas. Terms such as 'conceptual representation of reality' (Hazzard and Kergin, 1971) or 'Systematically constructed scientifically based and logically related set of concepts' (Johnson, 1975) do nothing to help the introduction of a formalized system of care into the accident and emergency setting.

The way forward

The Platt Report, *A Strategy for Nursing 1989* (Dept. of Health) provides the major lead in developing accident and emergency nursing into the 1990s and beyond. It identifies that within a changing world the nursing profession must change also, and recognizes that while change is never easy there must be changes in the nurses' attitudes and thinking. The report identifies the role of the nursing profession as first and foremost a response to human need. A greater emphasis must be placed on the dignity and autonomy of each individual; on the recognition of people as having ultimate responsibility for their own health and the right to full information about the choice which faces them. The targets for action include:

- Full accountability of nurses with the responsibility for individual patients should be recognized and applied in all health care settings.
- Development of primary nursing should be encouraged and new roles developed for nurses to improve care provision.
- Health education and promotion should become a major part of nursing care and views and wishes of the consumer must be taken into account.
- Standards must be set, research findings used in clinical practice and modern technology used to improve the quality of service provided.
- Nurses should accept responsibility for ensuring their own continued professional development and competency.

This document therefore provides the opportunity for nurses to progress in the development of philosophies of care within their specialty. Phrases such as individualized care, dignity, autonomy, self-care, patient information, nurses' accountability, health education and promotion must all be considered. It is a challenge not to be lost and the profession must not ignore this challenge.

Within the specialty of accident and emergency nursing, nurses need to identify in their own minds how they view the service and, more importantly, how they view the consumer of that service. In other words we must identify our beliefs and values; our philosophy regarding the service we provide and the consumers of that service, our fellow human beings. These philosophies, once they are identified, can then allow us to consider how the service can be structured and improved.

Identifying a philosophy for accident and emergency

Many of today's health care philosophies are very similar in content. They identify the fundamental rights of the individual as being paramount. Reflecting back to the Platt Report, *A Strategy for Nursing*, and the two major responsibilities of an accident and emergency department, it is clear that the philosophy must take account of the diversity of patients coming through the doors. The philosophy must also reflect the role of the nursing profession as identified in *A Strategy for Nursing* – to respond to human needs.

In the accident and emergency setting, all manner of human needs exist. They range from the sad and frightened child with a cut finger, to the bereaved parents who have just been told of their child's death; the drunk and violent patient on a Friday night to the elderly lady on a Sunday morning who can no longer cope at home. These patients all have very different needs and it is essential that any philosophy must contain the fundamental principles of treating each patient as an individual. The philosophy of the accident and emergency department therefore should be:

Nursing in accident and emergency is based on assisting the individual to maintain the two major values of life, health and quality of life. Each patient is an individual with individual human needs and as such, must retain their independence and dignity and have their freedom of choice and wishes taken into account. Each patient has the right to understand their treatment and care and for this care to be provided by skilled, nursing staff. The nurse, through a process of care, should encourage and assist the patient to remain independent and return to self-care as soon as possible. The medical, nursing, clerical and ancillary staff of the department, must work as a team to ensure that care provided for each patient allows these beliefs to be fostered. The environment of the department must be conducive to continual, educational development of the team and the retention of high standards of practice. To this end a process of care must be established. This process must be logically structured and contain a model of nursing and a triage system. It must be based on a problem orientated approach.

The process of care in accident and emergency

The process of care in accident and emergency must allow the nurse to return to looking at the patient and acting in response to her professional judgement, irrespective of the academic terminology. In other words a common-sense approach based on knowledge and skills. Validity and the reliability of the concepts that a nurse applies are the essence of her professional competence (Carnevali, 1973).

The process must comprise (Fig. 1/1):

1 A Model of Nursing.
2 A triage system.
3 A problem-orientated approach encompassing assessment, problem identification, goals, intervention and evaluation.
4 Documentation.

A MODEL OF NURSING

A Model of Nursing is simply a framework that provides a structure to nursing care. It is based on three essential elements:

1 Beliefs and values about human beings who are the recipients of nursing.
2 Achievable goals.
3 Knowledge and skill on which nursing practice is based.

(S. Wright, 1986) identifies it as simply a tool that helps nurses organize themselves. It organizes the nurses' thinking and provides orderly and logical practice. Pearson and Vaughan (1986) identify a nursing model as a picture or representation of what nursing actually is. Rambo (1984) defines it as a way of presenting a situation in logical terms to show the structure of the original idea or object.

Because accident and emergency nursing is primarily involved with the recognition and intervention of problems originating within a medical condition, it is easy to base care on a purely medical model and to forget that many of the problems identified may be specific to the individual's psychological, social and cultural background.

The medical model is based on the belief that man is a complex set of anatomical parts and physiological systems. Problems arise when there is a malfunction either within the anatomical part of the body or within a physiological system. Assessment is based on examination of the physiological and anatomical parts and care is aimed at restoring the body to normal function, either by the use of medication or surgery.

The great majority of patients seen in accident and emergency have a very specific physiological disturbance or anatomical injury. Therefore, within accident and emergency nursing, it is clearly ridiculous to ignore the medical model as a great deal of the nursing care is based on restoring normal anatomical and physiological activity. However, the use of a nursing model based on individual beliefs regarding the person as a whole is clearly more desirable as it allows the nurse to retain care of the physiological and anatomical parts, but also identify the human behavioural and social elements that may require intervention, e.g. bereavement counselling, environmental safety factors, psychological support, etc.

Many famous nurses have developed models of nursing. This in itself shows the range of nursing beliefs with regard to both humanity and our own profession. C. Roy presents a model based on four principle adaptation systems which influence behaviour. M. E. Rogers believes that humans are unitary fields of energy who interact as a whole with other energy fields within their environment. J. P. Riehl created an interactive model developed from a background of symbolic interactionist thought. (All three are cited in Aggleton and Chalmers (1984–5).)

Three major models of nursing that have become well known in the general nursing field are those developed by Henderson, Roper and Orem. V. Henderson (Aggleton and Chalmers, 1984–5) developed a model of nursing based on her belief that there are fourteen human needs: e.g. the need to breathe, eat, drink, eliminate, sleep, etc. She also defined nursing as primarily assisting the individual (sick or well) in the performance of those activities contributing to health or its recovery (or peaceful death) that (s)he would perform unaided if (s)he had the necessary strength, will or knowledge. The unique contribution of the nurse is to help the individual to be independent of such assistance as soon as possible.

N. Roper (Aggleton and Chalmers, 1984–5) developed her model from a model of living. It is based on her belief that humans have twelve activities of living and these in one form or other span from conception to death. Activities such as breathing, eating and drinking, communicating, mobilizing and maintaining a safe environment are all included.

Dorothy Orem first published her concept of nursing in 1959. A more formalized development of her model was initiated in 1965. Orem's Basic Structural Framework (1971) is based on her belief of humanity's need for self-care. In 1980 she defined self-care as the practice of activity that individuals initiate and perform on their own behalf in maintaining life, health and well-being. She identified nursing as giving direct assistance to a person unable to meet own self-care needs. The model is based on self-care demands. Six universal self-care demands are identified e.g. providing intake of air, water, food, control of excretion, etc. In ill health, Orem identifies three further self-care demands; these are termed health deviation self-care demands. Like all other models, each component interrelates with the other, so only for the purpose of description can they be separated. This separation can be related to a pattern or model of a car or dress. To function the object must be complete, but to achieve the end product a pattern must exist that identifies the various components required and facilitates the production of the item. In nursing the model is a whole thing, but to allow the use of the model for nursing care, the component parts must be identified. The model therefore allows for two major objectives to be achieved:

1 It provides the structure which allows for an organized approach to the assessment, planning, intervention and evaluation of patient care.
2 It retains the flexibility necessary for individualized nursing care of each patient.

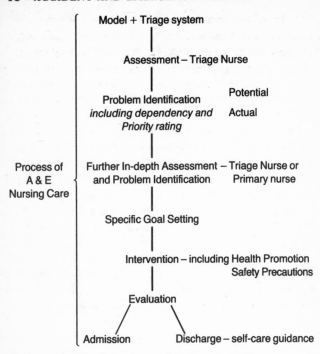

Fig. 1/1   A logical structured approach to A & E nursing

THE TRIAGE SYSTEM

Triage means to pick, sort, or select. It originates from the French word *trier* and has been used extensively throughout military medical history. The first reference to the word triage is found in the history of the English wool industry as early as 1727. During the 1800s it appeared in the coffee bean industry. In both, the selection and sorting of the product was described as triage. In Paris the triage point, a place or station, was used to sort out the good produce of the market from that to be thrown away. The first major use of triage in military history was seen in the First World War. It was used to sort out those casualties that could return to the battlefield and those who required limited medical resources. It also identified the salvageable from the non-salvageable patients. In mass casualty situations those patients who would probably live were dealt with immediately. Those who would probably die were left (delayed) until much later. As time progressed, the use of triage became more established and ordered. The triage point or station became not just a sorting point, but more a process unit. First Aid care was provided, patient flow was controlled and priority rating was based on a much improved patient assessment. Triage points became extended: the first in the field, the second at an evacuation area and a third at the hospital. Although in the field triage was still used to identify those patients who would need immediate hospitalization and those who were salvageable, the hospital triage point sorted into medical priorities on the basis that all patients were initially salvageable.

Modern-day triage

This is used in both the disaster situation and in the day-to-day running of the A & E Department.

Disaster triage

Disasters can be identified under two headings and two subheadings (Rutherford, 1989):

1 Simple disasters.
2 Compound disasters.

A simple disaster is where structures such as hospitals, roads, ambulances etc. are intact and available. A compound disaster is where, due to the nature of the disaster, these facilities are not available.

Compensated and uncompensated disasters A compensated disaster is where the casualty load is such that the medical capacity can cope. An uncompensated disaster is when it cannot.

The method of triage used must take the type of disaster into consideration. Most modern-day disasters are simple, compensated disasters and therefore the triage must be based on the philosophy that all patients that are alive are potentially salvageable. Priority ratings will be allocated on a 'need to transport' and a 'need for medical care' basis. Immediate, urgent and delayed (minor injuries) categories will be used. In a compound, uncompensated disaster, the same three triage categories will be used, but where patients are probably unsalvageable, despite their injuries, they will be placed in the delayed category.

Day-to-day accident and emergency triage

During a typical day triage is used by both the ambulance service personnel and the A & E staff. When dealing with a road-traffic accident affecting several patients the ambulance crew will determine the patient's priority order and transport the patients accordingly. On arrival in accident and emergency, a similar system of priority rating must exist ensuring the most seriously injured patient receives immediate medical care.

The first reference to the use of triage in A & E during a non-disaster situation, was in 1963 at Yale, Newhaven Hospital, USA. All patients when entering the A & E department were assessed by what was termed a Triage Officer. The Triage Officer was a physician. The physician assessed every patient on arrival in the emergency room and assigned an emergency rating. Since that day triage has developed and the Triage Officer has varied considerably ranging from physician, nurse, paramedic to Red Cross volunteer. Formal nurse triage in the UK appeared in the early 1980s. Today in both the USA and UK it is widely accepted that the most appropriate person to work as the Triage Officer is a qualified nurse with a wide experience and knowledge in the field of accident and emergency nursing.

Triage is seen now as an integral part of the process of A & E care. It sets the whole tone and pace of the patient's visit and ensures that all patients, irrespective of their mode of transport or apparent lack of injury, are seen by an experienced A & E nurse on arrival. Use of a properly organized triage system within A & E departments allows patients to be seen in priority order, not time order, and dispels the concept of 'first come first served'. It establishes a system of patient management which is clinically sound and far more reliable than traditional methods of patient reception. Although the true definition of triage is the sorting into groups of priorities, in contemporary use it encompasses many goals.

Goals of triage

1 Early patient assessment.
2 Priority rating
3 Assignment to correct area of care and infection control.
4 Control of patient flow.
5 Initiation of diagnostic measures.
6 Initiation of emergency care.
7 Patient education.

The most reliable method of achieving the above goals is to identify a triage nurse. The triage nurse using a model of nursing possesses the accepted beliefs, values, universal goals and the appropriate knowledge and skills to prioritize the patient properly, for both medical intervention and nursing care.

1 *Early patient assessment* The triage nurse uses a model of nursing as a tool to assess all patients presenting to the department. The assessment should not become lengthy otherwise a queue of patients will develop. Two factors determine the length of time the triage nurse should spend with each patient:

1 The presenting condition.
2 The number of patients to be triaged.

2 *Priority rating (the urgency of need)* The priority in which patients receive medical and nursing care depends on the identified problem following the nursing assessment. All patients who present to an accident and emergency department can crudely be categorized into two urgency ratings: urgent (priority one) or non-urgent (priority two). This two-category system has the disadvantage of allowing for too many patients to be placed in the non-urgent rating and the return of the 'first come, first served' philosophy.

In many accident and emergency departments, patients who

appear to have relatively minor injuries report to the reception desk and are categorized by the clerical staff into two groups. Group 1, those patients who are bleeding or collapsing at the reception desk; and group 2, all other patients. As most patients belong to group two, these people are sent by the clerk into the waiting room. A properly organized triage system removes the use of the clerical staff for prioritizing patients. This is clearly desirable and allows priority setting to be based on a formal nursing assessment.

3 *Assignment to correct area of care and infection control* During the assessment and priority rating stages the triage nurse will be deciding on the most appropriate area of care. Patients who require immediate life support will be allocated to the resuscitation room. Patients with a potential communicable disease will be placed into an isolation area and barrier nursing will be commenced. The majority of patients will be assigned to the waiting area until treatment can be provided. If the triage nurse is allowed by local health authority agreement to refer to other agencies, she may be assigning the patient direct to the GP, social work department, dentist, STD clinic, etc. If a nurse practitioner is working within the department, direct referral to this person may be the appropriate course of action.

4 *Control of patient flow* Patient allocation to correct areas of care can only occur if the triage nurse has control of all patient flow. The triage nurse must maintain a record of all trolley areas and be constantly aware of the current occupancy of all cubicles. Movement of patients from one area to another must be co-ordinated by this person. Many accident and emergency departments have more patients than cubicles available. Triage allows the most appropriate use of this valuable space.

5 *Initiation of diagnostic measures* Following the assessment stage the nurse often identifies certain diagnostic measures that will be necessary to allow the doctor to make a full diagnosis. X-ray is one diagnostic measure where if the nurse is permitted by the health authority to send the patient to X-ray the patient's waiting time can

be reduced quite considerably. Other examples are the recording of an ECG and the ordering of relevant blood tests.

6 *Initiation of emergency care* Although triage is strictly related to the sorting and prioritizing of patients, it is inevitable that the triage nurse will provide some form of emergency care. This care will vary depending on the individual. Lifting of the jaw to provide an open airway in the unconscious patient would be appropriate care during the assessment stage. The application of temporary dressings, slings and splints are other forms of emergency care which the triage nurse will perform. The removal of a sub-tarsal foreign body from the patient's eye is another area where the triage nurse is preventing further injury while the patient awaits the medical or nurse practitioner's treatment.

7 *Patient education* A major part of the triage nurse's job is health promotion and advice on safety. Many patients present to accident and emergency because their understanding of self-care is limited. During the assessment the nurse can identify a number of areas where advice will prevent further visits. Self-care instruction on discharge also enables the patient to retain independence and return to health.

THE PROBLEM-ORIENTATED APPROACH

The majority of patients presenting to the accident and emergency department complain of a particular problem, e.g. cut finger, ankle injury or multiple injuries following a road or industrial accident. Many other actual and potential problems can be identified following a full nursing assessment. By using the model of nursing and the triage system, the nurse can assess, identify actual and potential problems, set realistic goals, carry out intervention and evaluate the care given. This problem-orientated approach using the accident and emergency model and triage system, provides a logical, systematic delivery of nursing care.

Assessment

Nursing assessment should be the first stage in the total provision of individualized care, tailored to suit the needs of each individual patient. The nursing assessment should take place as soon after the patient enters the department as possible. The patient who walks into the department should be offered the same provision for immediate assessment as the patient suffering multiple injuries. This will occur if the triage system has been organized correctly. Nursing assessment, when carried out by an experienced A & E nurse, allows for correct identification of problems and appropriate intervention.

Identifying actual and potential problems

Analysis of the data collected during the assessment stage enables the nurse to identify all problems clearly. Some problems will be obvious, e.g. a compound fracture with the bone protruding through the skin. Other actual problems may be less obvious, e.g. the loss of will to live. Potential problems are those that are not present at the time of arrival but may occur at a later stage. A patient with a wrist fracture may develop an obstruction to the blood flow. An elderly patient who is immobile will develop pressure sores; if appropriate, preventative care is provided. Some problems will need immediate intervention, others can safely wait.

Goal-setting and intervention

The nurse must state a specific result which should be achievable. The universal goals of nursing in A & E which must be identified, during the development stage of the model, will act as guidance for the development of specific goals relating to each individual patient. Intervention must allow for the goals that are set to be achieved. The intervention stage of the process, will, like the assessment stage, be based on the components of the model used.

Evaluation

This final step in the process of care is essential. Evaluation allows for the identification of goals that have been achieved and others that may have not. New problems may also be identified, the nursing care plan may require alteration to meet the new or original needs. When evaluating, the nurse must always consider:

1 Were the goals logical? Were they achievable?
2 Has intervention taken place as required?

DOCUMENTING THE PROCESS OF CARE

The process of care in accident and emergency must be in your head. The process itself is how you think patient care. By thinking through the components of your model, and taking the care process step by step, the achievement of a logical, structured approach to your nursing care will exist. Documenting that process is important, but it should not create mountains of paper. Nursing records are essential. They form a legal document. An education tool. They provide guidance and instruction for the actual delivery of nursing care. The DHSS circular PL/CNO(88) 17 draws attention to the need for accurate and detailed nursing records. It identifies that nursing records are visible evidence of the care given and the circular requests action to be taken to ensure nursing records are maintained and a system of monitoring is introduced.

In the A & E department a method must be devised that does not slow down the process of medical and nursing care. It must be useable in a department seeing 50–60 patients a day, as well as in one that deals with 200 patients a day. It must be able to record all parts of the care from assessment to evaluation.

TAKING THE PROCESS A STAGE FURTHER

Change for change's sake is never a good philosophy. Developing the structured approach to patient care is not so much a change as a tidying up of the current care system. Milne suggested that the

the more things change, the more they stay the same. In some situations this may be true. But I would like to believe that by developing and documenting the process of care, things do not stay the same, and that nurses are helped to make nursing better. The process of care can go hand in hand with other developments taking place in the accident and emergency specialty. Primary nursing and the nurse practitioner allow the process to be taken forward in the clinical setting. The process of care also provides the golden opportunity to develop a true clinical career structure for nurses.

Primary nursing

Primary nursing has four design elements:

1 The allocation and acceptance of individual responsibility for decision-making to one individual.
2 Individual assignment of patient care.
3 Direct communication channels.
4 One person responsible for the quality of care administered to the patient throughout the total care period.

The primary nurse accepts three major responsibilities:

1 To collect information, including research findings, needed to care for her patients and make it available to colleagues.
2 To assess the patient and produce a written plan of action and criteria for evaluation.
3 To accept responsibility for planning and co-ordinating the patient's discharge.

Analysis of the design elements and major responsibilities of primary nursing, suggests that to some extent, it is taking place in many accident and emergency departments today. Unfortunately what is not happening is nurses becoming true specialists. Many accident and emergency nurses despite working in the specialty for many years, do not become accident and emergency nurse specialists. They have not identified the necessary research, they do not always plan their activity or evaluation correctly and do not always accept the total nursing responsibility for the patient. Care of a patient in accident and emergency can still become fragmented, with several nurses being involved with the provision of care and the responsibility for all patient care still being held by the nurse in charge. If accident and emergency nurses are going to become prime care providers they must personally take the major responsibility for the care of one or a group of patients in the A & E setting.

They must plan and implement programmes of care. The individual nurse must be responsible for that patient's care from admission to discharge, even though delivery of care can be assigned to another nurse.

Advantages of developing the primary nursing system in A & E

1 The patient develops a partnership with one nurse.
2 Clear documentation by the major care provider ensures continuation of care.
3 The primary nurse is accountable and therefore is encouraged to develop clinical skills, leadership and interpersonal skills.
4 Communication improves.
5 Quality assessment is made easier.

Disadvantages
The disadvantages of such a system can include:

1 Stress on the primary nurse.
2 Associate nurses may become demoralized.
3 Patient and nurse may not get on.

Making the change
The move to primary nursing in the accident and emergency setting should be easier than in the ward. Already many patients have an identified nurse to provide care throughout the stay in accident and emergency, e.g. the multiply injured patient. Others could easily be afforded this facility. The nurse in charge of the department would become more of a co-ordinator and resource person. The major change is with nurses themselves. Nurses who work in accident and emergency must recognize that to become a specialist does not simply mean spending years in accident and emergency. It means

constantly developing and understanding the specialty. It means being accountable for decisions, planning, intervention and evaluation of patient care. It means following a logically developed process of care.

Nurse practitioner

A nurse practitioner in accident and emergency is a nurse specialist with additional skills in physical diagnosis, psychosocial assessment, the prescribing of care, preventative treatment and the promotion of health. The nurse practitioner is available to members of the public who present with health problems. The role allows for autonomous decisions to be made regarding the initial assessment of the patient and if necessary referral to other agencies to achieve overall patient care. The patient always retains the right of choice between seeing the nurse practitioner or the doctor, and better communication between the service and the individual will exist.

In the majority of cases the nurse practitioner, having made a nursing diagnosis, will provide treatment and discharge the patient. Many minor injuries can be dealt with by the nurse practitioner and this prevents unnecessary waiting times for many patients. In addition to this advantage the nurse practitioner is able to reduce the number of inappropriate attenders by offering health advice. Nurse practitioners can also provide comprehensive follow-up care, certain counselling skills and a more rapid referral system. The nurse practitioner should be trained to enable her to acquire the knowledge and skills to carry out the role. The training should enable the nurse to make a clinical assessment or diagnosis based upon the history or physical examination of the minor illness or injury attended. A logical plan of care to manage the patient's health problems can be drawn up and if necessary, appropriate follow-up care arranged.

The training curriculum for the nurse practitioner should be based on four modules:

1 Assessment and diagnosis.
2 Treatment and prescribing.

3 Communication skills.
4 Health behaviour and prevention of illness and injury.

The nurse practitioner role should not be seen as a substitute for the A & E doctor, but as a further development of the holistic approach to patient care in the A & E setting.

Summary

Nursing in accident and emergency, because of the rapid inter-action between nurse and patient, can become uncoordinated. The process of care is not new, it merely acts as a vehicle for delivering nursing care in an organized and structured manner. A model of nursing provides a framework. It allows nurses to work together without practising in conflicting ways. It allows them to share ideas and thoughts concerning their beliefs about people, their goals, and to develop the knowledge on which they base their practice.

The triage system allows the model to be used in a structured way to provide rapid assessment of all patients. To identify the problems and organize goals, intervention and evaluation. Documentation of the nursing care is essential:

> 'I do not pretend to teach her how. I ask her to
> teach herself, and for this purpose, I venture to
> give her some hints.'
>
> Florence Nightingale, 1860

2 *A model of nursing for accident and emergency*

The decision to use a particular model of nursing, or a combination of models must be made at departmental level. Factors that influence this choice are:

1 The philosophy of the department.
2 Current nursing practice within the department.
3 The need for the model to be easily memorized and recalled.
4 The need for flexibility in its use.
5 The need for the model to lend itself to easy documentation.

Within general nursing today many wards have successfully implemented the models created by Henderson, Roper and Orem. The systematic approach these models allow has provided many nurses with the tool required to achieve a structured approach to patient assessment and subsequent care. The question therefore is can one or a combination of these models be successfully used in the A & E setting or is there a need for a totally new model to be developed? Analysis of the three models (Henderson, Roper and Orem) shows that:

1 The fourteen needs (Henderson), twelve activities of living (Roper) and six universal self-care demands (Orem) all cover the same major life requirements (Tables 2/1–2/3).
2 The need for care to be provided on an individualized basis is paramount.
3 People need independence. Henderson identifies the nurse as performing activities for the individual, only because the patient cannot perform them unaided. The nurse is helping the individual to independence. Roper's model is based on maintaining or restoring independence in activities and avoiding ill-health by independent, preventative measures. Orem bases her model on the total concept of self-care.

4 The underlying philosophy within the Platt report *A Strategy for Nursing* and my own philosophy for accident and emergency is clearly reflected within the three models.

Table 2/1   Henderson's fundamental needs

  1 Breathe normally.
  2 Eat and drink adequately.
  3 Eliminate body waste.
  4 Move and maintain desirable posture.
  5 Sleep and rest.
  6 Select suitable clothes – dress and undress.
  7 Maintain body temperature within normal range.
  8 Keep the body clean and well groomed and protect the skin.
  9 Avoid dangers in the environment and avoid injuring others.
 10 Communicate with others expressing emotions, needs, fears or opinions.
 11 Worship according to one's faith.
 12 Work in such a way that there is a sense of accomplishment.
 13 Play or participate in various forms of recreation.
 14 Learn, discover or satisfy the curiosity that leads to normal development and health and use the available health facilities.

Table 2/2   Roper's activities of daily living

  1 Maintaining a safe environment.
  2 Breathing.
  3 Eliminating.
  4 Controlling body temperature.
  5 Working and playing.
  6 Sleeping.
  7 Communicating.
  8 Eating and drinking.
  9 Personal cleansing and dressing.
 10 Mobilizing.
 11 Expressing sexuality.
 12 Dying.

Table 2/3   Orem's universal self-care needs

  1 Sufficient intake of air, water, nutrition.
  2 Satisfactory elimination functions.
  3 Activity balanced with rest.
  4 Time spent alone balanced with time spent with others.
  5 Prevention of danger to self.
  6 Being 'normal'.

Current nursing practice

Current nursing practice in accident and emergency highlights key components such as communication and support of major physiological activities of the body e.g. breathing, circulation, mobility. It reflects the belief that humans are individuals with individual human needs and encourages them to return to independence, supported by health education, self-care guidance on discharge and, if necessary, service within the community.

CHOOSING THE MODEL

From this analysis of the three models and observation of current nursing practice it would appear that any one of the three models could possibly be used in the A & E setting. However, if it is accepted that for a model to work in accident and emergency it needs to be in our minds and in the way we think, then clearly all three have shortcomings. Henderson's model requires the nurse to be familiar with fourteen needs of the patient. Using the Roper model requires twelve activities of living to be considered. Orem's model requires six universal self-care demands and three health deviancy demands to be memorized and recalled when used for patient assessment.

Nursing documentation of all these models can become lengthy, and delays in patient care could occur. What is required is a model that can be used in any A & E department, however busy and varied in its patient throughput. It must be suitable for use with the patient suffering a minor injury as well as the patient with a major medical, surgical or traumatic condition. It must be based on the concept of individualized human needs and the needs for independence and self-care. It must lend itself to easy recall and documentation.

Developing a much simpler model

Nursing models can be developed in two ways:

1 The theorist may conceive an idea, expound and develop it into a model, then put it into practice.
2 Practice itself can be analysed and the model developed to represent what actually exists.

When considering the possibility of developing a simple model for use in the A & E department, it is clear that the creation of a totally new model of nursing is unnecessary. It is also apparent from the observation of nursing practice, that parts of nursing models are in use. The philosophy of self-care and independence is present. There appears to be an underlying belief regarding the individual.

Any nursing model must be able to integrate with the medical model. Just as nursing and medical staff work closely together in A & E, so must the models. In fact the accident and emergency model could be visualized as a nursing model encompassing the core of the medical model (Fig. 2/1). This concept may shock some nursing academics, but in accident and emergency, it is reality. The majority of patients attending the accident and emergency department are suffering from a defect of an anatomical part or a disruption of a physiological system. Therefore nurses are working with a medical model, *but* by using an accident and emergency model of nursing, the care goes beyond the anatomical or physiological problem and identifies all the individual problems. Care is then provided accordingly. This then is where we begin.

Building the model

Like any other model of nursing, my accident and emergency model is developed logically. It contains three essential elements:

1 Beliefs and values about human beings as the recipients of care in accident and emergency.
2 Achievable goals.
3 Knowledge and skill on which nursing practice is based.

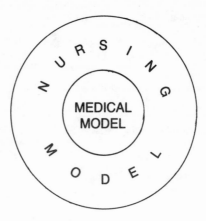

Fig. 2/1 The nursing model encompassing the core of the medical model

BELIEF AND VALUES

The model, like my philosophy for the accident and emergency department, is based on the belief that humans are individuals with individual human needs. It is based also on the belief that during their life-span the individual is engaged in various self-care activities in an attempt to retain independence. Seven components of life comprising physical, human behavioural and social aspects can be identified which must be kept in appropriate balance to maintain health and quality of life. Due an event (physical or mental illness or injury) in the course of the individual's life-span, the balance between the various components can become upset and the ability to maintain health and quality of life will be disrupted.

The individual identifies the accident and emergency staff as the resource to assist them in the re-balance of the components of life, re-establishment of independence and thus a continuation of physical, emotional and social comfort.

The seven components of life can be clearly identified (Fig. 2/2). The reasoning behind these is given below. Their practical consequences for the A & E nurse are detailed on pages 34–9.

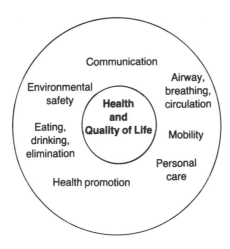

Fig. 2/2   Physical, human behavioural and social components of life

1 Communication

Humans are social beings who through communication and relationship with others achieve quality of life. Partnership is developed through communication and information is shared. Communication can be verbal or non-verbal. Different modes of human behaviour due to attitude, religious beliefs, moods, sexual identity and emotion are all expressed by communication. The five physiological senses – sight, hearing, taste, smell and touch – allow us to communicate with the world. Pain is communicated to us and between us in many different ways.

2 Airway, breathing and circulation

Oxygen is vital to life. To ensure normal tissue activity, a clear airway, normal respiratory function and adequate circulating blood volume is essential. Oxygen is used in the metabolic process of energy and body temperature is maintained. Loss of any of these functions will lead to ill-health.

3 Mobility

Our ability to move enables us to engage in various activities at work and play. It allows the individual to accomplish various tasks to maintain independence and achieve quality of life. Mobility relies on a functional musculoskeletal system.

4 Environmental safety

Safety within the environment is a key factor. Depending on the individual's work, lifestyle and attitude, the degree of risk will vary. Self-care normally results in the appropriate safety measures being taken. The individual's living environment can constitute a risk to health, unless additional safety measures are taken.

5 Personal care

Good hygiene can minimize the spread of infection and attention to personal cleanliness will affect the individual's health. The individual's ability to maintain personal care can be influenced by physical and psychosocial illness.

6 Eating, drinking and elimination

Health can only be maintained with adequate intake of food and water. This enables normal body function to continue. Waste products of metabolism are eliminated from the body.

7 Health promotion

Humans have the desire to remain in good health. Economic as well as social circumstances have a bearing on health. To achieve good health we often require others to maintain a clean environment. There is conflict between the desire for health, and social activities which put health at risk. A balance has to be achieved and this depends very much on how highly the individual rates his own self-care in health promotion.

Goals of accident and emergency nursing

WHAT THE NURSE AIMS TO ACHIEVE

Four universal goals can be identified which relate to all patients in the accident and emergency setting. Following patient assessment, specific goals for each individual can also be identified.

UNIVERSAL GOALS

1 To establish a partnership with the patient/relatives.
2 To achieve a level of independence in the patient appropriate to his condition or injury and by so doing, assist him to restore health and quality of life.
3 To enable the individual to avoid ill-health or injury through self-care, health education and environmental safety.
4 To ensure that optimum effectiveness of medically prescribed treatment is obtained.

1 Establishing a partnership with the patient

Partnership is established through communication. Both parties need to be committed to the establishment of a partnership role.

Nursing can only exist when a partnership has been formed between the individual and the nurse. The patient who rejects this relationship will find difficulty in appreciating the process of care and need for self-care guidance. The nurse must attempt to prevent her attitude or prejudice influencing the establishment of the partnership and causing a breakdown in communication.

The nurse, through a programme of education, must develop communication skills and interview techniques. The ability to listen and react appropriately to emotional responses of the patients/ relatives is essential. The nurse must have a working knowledge of sociological aspects of family culture, social class, etc. in relation to health. An understanding of altered body image, mental health, the specific needs of children and human behaviour is also necessary. The skill in identifying and alleviating pain is essential.

2   Achieving a level of independence in the patient

Most models of nursing have built into them the concept of the patient's need for independence. The nurse must identify the degree of independence and set the goal appropriate to the patients' condition. Although independence is desirable, some patients will have total dependency on the nurse. Others will have some degree of independence, but will either require support, treatment or assistance to re-establish full independence or will never regain full independence and will require support in the community/hospital from nurses and other health care professionals (Fig. 2/3).

The nurse, during the assessment stage of the process of care, must use her knowledge of physiology and potential disorders of the various systems of the body, to assist in the identification of problems and setting of specific goals. She must be aware of the importance of base-line observation and vital signs. Specifically she should be able to recognize problems with the airway, breathing and circulation, including recognition of shock. The nurse should be aware of the causes of vomiting and effect of illness or injury on the gastro-intestinal system and urinary system. She should be able to assess the major functions of the musculoskeletal system and identify any abnormalities. The nurse must have acquired the

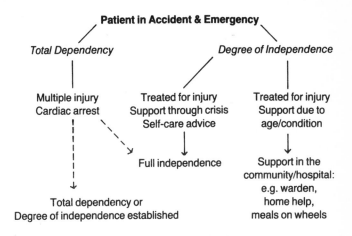

Fig. 2/3   Patient dependency in A & E

relevant knowledge and be proficient in her intervention skills to enable her to intervene appropriately and achieve the goals set, especially relating to life support.

3 Avoiding ill-health/injury through self-care or preventative measures

The individual's lifestyle and attitude to self-care in health will determine the ability to avoid preventable ill-health or injury. The nurse in accident and emergency must strive to assist the patient with self-care. Health education and advice on safety within the individual's environment will avoid further visits to the accident and emergency department. The nurse must have acquired a knowledge of health promotion and the appropriate skills required to convey the message to the patient. The nurse should be aware of health education material, the role of public health, health promotion departments and screening systems. The nurse should have a working knowledge of the Health and Safety at Work Act and be aware of safety factors in the home and within the A & E department. She should have a knowledge of environmental safety aspects, especially relating to the elderly patient.

4 Obtaining optimum effectiveness of medically prescribed treatment

The majority of patients seen in the A & E department require medical intervention. The nurse, apart from identifying and providing nursing care, must ensure that the patient obtains the best from the medical treatment. Correct care of the suture wound will allow the wound to heal. Medication taken in the correct dose, at the correct time, will assist the patient to overcome his ill-health. Self-care guidance is often essential for the patient, allowing the full benefit of medical care to be achieved.

The nurse must have gained knowledge of the action of medication and possible side-effects. The process of wound healing and possible infection risks should be known. Skills relating to support of medical treatment must be acquired, e.g. the nurse's role in the care of the patient and equipment during a chest drain insertion.

Knowledge and skills

Just as the universal goals of accident and emergency nursing relate to the beliefs and values, so the knowledge and skills required by the A & E nurse must relate to the stated goals.

Carnevali (1973) noted that the knowledge that a nurse uses in a nursing situation is at least as important as the action taken.

Much of the knowledge and skills will be acquired through in-service training and ongoing development of the nurse in the specialty of accident and emergency nursing. Many national board courses are relevant to the A & E specialty, including the Accident & Emergency Course, the Accident and Emergency Advanced

Course, Care of Violent or Potentially Violent Patient, The Teaching and Assessment Course, and Care of Children and the Elderly in Accident and Emergency. The Accident and Emergency trained nurse must maintain a high degree of knowledge and skill, based on sound research.

Making the model work

The beliefs, values, universal goals, knowledge and skills have been established. The model can now be used in the A & E setting to provide the logical structure required to enable patient care to take place. Using the seven components of life as the tool, a full assessment of the individual will lead to problems being identified, specific goals being set and intervention taking place in sequential priority order. Each component of life should be considered as a piece of a jigsaw. All components must be assessed by the nurse. A first stage – non-written assessment – can be performed with a second, more detailed stage – recorded. Not all components will require intervention. By identifying the components that require intervention, the nurse can organize a logical nursing care plan to achieve the set goals. Dependency rating and the setting of priorities (triage) will be made much simpler.

USING THE COMPONENTS OF LIFE

Having introduced the seven components of life, for easy recall, and because of the close relationships between health promotion and environmental safety, these two components can be combined.

In daily use, therefore, six life components can be recalled during any stage of the care process (Fig. 2/4):

1 Communication (developing the partnership):
   (a) Personal details, name, age, etc.
   (b) History.
   (c) Chief complaint.
   (d) Conscious level.

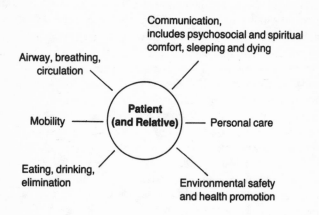

Fig. 2/4   Using the components of life

    (e) Human behaviour pattern.
    (f) Physiological senses.
2 Airway, breathing, circulation (body temperature).
3 Mobility:
    (a) Individual limbs.
    (b) The whole body.
4 Personal care.
5 Eating, drinking and elimination.
6 Environmental safety and health promotion.

Communication

Before care can normally get underway, communication must exist so the partnership is established. Janis (1971) records that hospitalization, like many other stressful events, produces a sharp increase in our need for social reassurance, particularly from relatives and the professional personnel responsible for care. Through communication, the nurse will obtain a full history of the reason for the visit to accident and emergency. The nurse will often need to take most of the initiative at the early stage to create a harmonious relationship with the patient and relatives. Observation of the patient's position, ability to walk and facial expression can communicate a number of non-verbal signs. Pain will often be expressed in this way, as will aggression. Unconscious patients can achieve some form of communication and the nurse should always talk to such patients. The human behaviour of both the nurse and patient will affect the establishment of good communication. Drugs and alcohol can create a barrier to an effective partnership developing. This problem can be seen regularly in many A & E departments and can often lead to violence towards staff. All nursing staff must develop communication skills in relation to children. Written information should be duplicated.

During the assessment stage specific problems can be identified and recorded. Intervention under the communication component will include such nursing care as bereavement support, correct positioning of the patient to reduce pain, listening to the patient and supporting the patient emotionally and spiritually when required. Intervention for disturbed patients will also be included under this component as will any disorder affecting the physiological senses.

Airway, breathing and circulation

A, B, C. These are the most essential letters to remember.

Airway – A clear airway is essential for life. The normal passage of gases between the outside air and alveoli must occur. The nurse must ensure a clear airway in present and any obstruction to the airway is cleared immediately.

Breathing – The ability to exchange gases relies on normal, respiratory function. The nurse must assess any defect in this function and intervene as necessary. Increased oxygen intake may be required. Neurological or mechanical defects will lead to problems with respiration.

Circulation – Any reduction in the pump mechanism or vascular tree will have a direct effect on the patient's ability to maintain normal metabolism, energy and temperature. Loss of body fluid reduces the ability to transport essential products round the body. Assessment of the cardiovascular state will identify problems and the essential intervention required, e.g. pressure bandages to stop haemorrhage. Peripheral pulses, distal to limb injuries and cardio-respiratory arrest, should also be included under this component. Care of the airway, breathing or circulation, takes priority over any other nursing action.

Mobility

Reduction in mobility will vary considerably between age groups and the injury sustained. The young footballer will be less restricted in his activities following an ankle injury than an elderly person living alone. The footballer, even with the use of crutches, would still be able to go to the local pub with his team. The elderly person may not even be able to move from the chair. The loss of mobility can greatly affect the socializing activity of life, which is important for psychological stability. The ability to sit up from a lying position, or rise and walk from a chair, gives an indication as to the patient's ability to cope at home. The use of walking aids, splints and other support aids, should be included in this component.

Personal care

Assessing the patient's clothing, skin condition and body odour often provides the information on personal care. Conditions in the home, ill health or the individual's behaviour can lead to a decrease in the patient's ability to perform personal care. Intervention may take the form of advice, support and perhaps even providing the patient with a shower or wash in the A & E department. Responsibility for the safe custody of valuables and clothing, should also be considered under this heading.

Eating, drinking and elimination

Adequate fluids and nutrition must be taken to sustain life. In the A & E department both are normally restricted, especially in the injured. Information regarding the last intake of food or fluid is often essential for care in A & E to continue. Diabetic patients will require blood sugar monitoring to be performed in accident and emergency. Patients will often present to A & E suffering a change in elimination. Elimination of urine may be obstructed and abnormal bowel movement can lead to severe dehydration. Elimination of stomach content especially in the unconscious patient, requires immediate intervention to prevent airway obstruction. Patients who have taken an overdose of drugs will be encouraged to eliminate the stomach contents.

Environmental safety and health promotion

Environmental safety can be considered under three sub-headings:

1 Is the patient/relative safe in the work place or home environment?
2 Is the patient safe to return to work or home environment?
3 Is the environment within the A & E department safe?

Patients will injure themselves at home or work, either due to inadequate safety precautions or inadequate use of safety device. The home can be very unsafe for the young or old. The tablets that look like smarties, the rug on a polished floor. When assessing patients the nurse should consider all the possible environmental factors which may have caused the injury or illness and through intervention, encourage environmental safety. Many patients have dependent relatives at home e.g. elderly parents or children. Without supervision they could be environmentally unsafe. Nurses must make adequate arrangements for such dependents, thus ensuring their safety.

The patient in the department must be safe. Use of trolley sides and adequate observation will help. Identification of dependency also has a bearing on environmental safety. Does the patient understand instructions? A patient with diminished responsibility due to injury, illness or an inbuilt deficit, may be at risk if left unattended, purely because of their inability to comply with the request not to leave the trolley or the room. The isolation of patients who may have a communicable disease also ensures the safety of staff and other patients.

Many opportunities arise in the accident and emergency department to promote health education. These can range from information in the waiting room to specific one-to-one discussions with the patient. The patients can be advised on methods of preventing ill-health or the best way to treat any further injury e.g. next time it is better not to put butter on the burn.

Parents can be guided in the prevention of febrile convulsions in the child and the patients with respiratory disorders can be advised on the need to stop smoking. Self-care guidance following treatment should be considered under this component. Correct care of the wound can prevent infection occurring. Correct care of the sprained ankle will allow the patient to become independent as rapidly as possible.

HELPING THE STAFF TO WORK WITH THE MODEL

As with any new development, staff will require help with the use of the model, thereby achieving the best results from its implementation. A more detailed diagram (Fig. 2/5) of the key components with sub-headings can be displayed within the department. This allows the nurse to familiarize herself with the various items under each heading.

USING THE MODEL WITH TRIAGE

The model having been developed specifically to provide a more structured approach to patient care can obviously be used during triage. The nurse will assess the patient's components of life and be in a much stronger position to determine the priority rating and patient dependency. This next stage in the process of care, therefore, relies on a well-established triage system.

History, Conscious State, Verbal and Non-verbal Communication, Pain.
Human Behaviour – attitude, religious beliefs, mood, emotion, effect of drugs
                   and alcohol.
                 – response to sudden death and support of bereaved
                   relatives.
Physical Senses – sight, hearing, taste, smell, touch.

EATING, DRINKING, ELIMINATION
Food/fluid intake
Bowels, bladder problems
Vomiting
Reason for nil by mouth
Naso-gastric tubes
Catheters
Blood sugar levels

Patient (and Relative)

AIRWAY, BREATHING, CIRCULATION
Airway – assessment of care
Breathing – assessment of respiratory
            function
          – chest movement
          – care of patients with
            respiratory problem
Circulation – assessment of central
              and peripheral
              circulation
            – care of patients with
              wounds
            – cardiac disorders
            – external and internal
              haemorrhage
            – I.V. fluids
Metabolism – temperature changes

MOBILITY
All muscular/skeletal problems
All assessment and intervention
required
Mobility, activity, work and play
Assessment and intervention regarding
relevant mobility due to age
Use of splints, walking aids, etc.

PERSONAL CARE
Cleanliness
Washing, bathing
– ability
Clothes – state of

ENVIRONMENTAL SAFETY & HEALTH PROMOTION
Safe Accident & Emergency environment
Isolation of patients with communicable diseases
Safety in the home – lack of
Safety in the workplace – lack of
Independent lifestyle and attitude to safety and health
Facilities at home for the disabled/elderly: e.g. warden,
bath rails, etc.
Information on safety and health

Fig. 2/5   The seven components of life

Summary

Despite a number of nursing models currently being used within nursing today, a much simpler model is necessary for use in the Accident and Emergency department. The model must achieve certain criteria:

1 It must reflect the philosophy of the department.
2 It must reflect current nursing practice in the department.
3 It must be easily memorized and recalled.
4 It must be flexible.
5 It must be easily documented.

The model that has been recommended achieves all the above. It is based on the belief that humans are individuals with specific human needs and each individual is engaged in self-care activities. The model identifies seven components of life which must be kept in appropriate balance to maintain health and quality of life.

The model can be used within the accident and emergency department to give a more structured approach to the problem-orientated method of delivering nursing care. Each component can be assessed by the nurse and problems identified. Intervention can be provided under the same component headings and evaluation is made easier.

3 Developing the triage system

As indicated in the introductory chapter, triage should be used in the A & E department during a typical working day and should not only be implemented during a major incident. A well-organized triage system is crucial to the process of A & E care and allows full use of the A & E model of nursing.

Problems to be addressed

One of the first considerations to be made when developing a triage system is the need for discussion with, and support from, all members of the A & E team. Although triage has become a familiar word within A & E nursing circles, the concept of triage may be quite new to many of the staff. A number of nurses and doctors still consider triage to be the duty of the receptionist. Conflict can exist between medical and nursing staff. Many doctors do not approve, nor can they even contemplate nurses officially making decisions regarding the priority in which they will see patients – even though this happens daily. Nurses themselves have difficulty with the question of accountability and their legal and professional position when making decisions as to who should wait and who must be seen.

The receptionists inevitably will feel hurt, they may jump to the conclusion that all the years of working in the A & E department and the experience in knowing who to take in and who to leave in the waiting-room, is being dismissed as irrelevant.

Time must be spent on explaining the advantages of triage without condemning past practice. Triage addresses the increased expectations of patients. It allows the nurse to see the patient early on in his or her care. It creates an environment conducive to the provision of a high-quality service. Reference to easy reading on triage will help your colleagues. Photo-copy recent articles, but choose carefully, you do not want to put them off the idea. Organize lunchtime workshops to allow all staff to participate in the planning stage, but have a small planning team who will see the implement-ation through. The consultant, senior nurse manager, sister and staff nurse should be sufficient. It must be made clear that the receptionist does not become redundant. The receptionist will still be required to complete registration of all patients. If the triage nurse is attending to a patient and another patient enters the department in a collapsed state, the receptionist should still sum-mon aid immediately. Depending on the system of triage adopted, it may still be necessary, though not ideal, for the receptionist to divert some patients to one area and some to another area.

Accountability

The triage nurse is accountable for the decisions made regarding triage. It is essential, therefore, that only a nurse who has completed local training and has been found competent to assess, identify problems and prioritize patients should be working at the triage area. The nurse does not make a medical diagnosis but formulates an accurate clinical impression, based on her knowledge. The nurse should be able to show that with the use of the A & E model a complete and comprehensive assessment has been made and the patient prioritized and allocated an appropriate area in the department.

THE PATIENT WHO DIES IN THE WAITING-ROOM –
WHO IS AT FAULT?

This situation can and does occur. The area of negligence will depend very much on the triage nurse's assessment. Example – a patient presents with chest pains. The assessment is as follows:

1 Communication – painful chest muscles last week, only when moving the arm.

2 History of heavy manual work, prior to pain.
3 A.B.C. all stable.
4 Skin colour normal.
5 Temperature normal.
6 No other complaint.

If the patient suddenly has a cardiac arrest in the waiting-room it is not reasonable to hold the triage nurse responsible. If however, the assessment had clearly suggested that the pain could have been of cardiac origin, then the nurse would have been at fault had the patient been prioritized to a low category and been left in the waiting-room.

Setting up the system

Once the decision to go ahead with triage has been made and all staff are willing to work on a pilot scheme, the next process is setting up the system. A triage policy must be established and procedures and protocols formulated. The policy must include guidelines on the degree of assessment to be carried out by the triage nurse. It must also include the priority rating system.

Training programmes need to be organized so all staff are carrying out triage in a similar manner.

DEGREE OF ASSESSMENT

By identifying the workload of the department the activity of the triage nurse can be anticipated. The nurse may have time to undertake in-depth patient assessment, or due to the throughput may only have time to identify the chief complaint and carry out a 90-second survey. The patient's condition from initial observation by the triage nurse will also influence the assessment time. Patients who are brought into the department unconscious or apparently seriously injured will require a rapid 90-second assessment. This assessment includes the identification of the communication component – e.g. Is the patient conscious or unconscious? – and the airway, breathing and circulation component – e.g. check airway, check breathing, check patient's major pulses. Observe patient's skin colour and any obvious major blood loss from external wounds. Patients with life-threatening conditions will be taken to the resuscitation area, and the primary nurse will continue the assessment at this stage.

Patients with less serious injuries can spend a longer period with the triage nurse, and a much fuller assessment can take place. Old records can also be requested and the partnership can develop between the patient and nurse so an identifiable care giver is recognized by the patient during the waiting period.

PRIORITY RATING SYSTEM (FIG. 3/1)

The simplest system, but not the most effective, is the two-category priority system. Priority one includes all patients who need immediate or urgent care. Priority two includes all other patients. It is clear that many patients in priority two will have varying degrees of need and consequently a priority system with more categories is desirable. A three-rating system provides more flexibility: immediate (priority one), urgent (priority two) and delayed (priority three). Further subdivisions of these headings can lead to a five or six rating scale. I recommend the four-category rating scale.

Patient { Urgent — Priority 1
Non-urgent — Priority 2

Patient { Immediate — Priority 1
Urgent — Priority 2
Delay — Priority 3

Patient { Immediate — Priority 1
Urgent — Priority 2
Semi-urgent — Priority 3
Delay — Priority 4
No need for care — Priority 5

Fig. 3/1 Priority rating

THE FOUR-CATEGORY RATING SCALE (FIG. 3/2)

With four categories to choose from, the nurse has a much more flexible tool in triage than with any other category rating system. Less than four can lead to a large percentage of patients being allocated the delay category, or inappropriate patients being allocated the Urgent category. More than four categories can lead to unnecessary confusion and difficulty with implementation. The four-category scale consists of:

1 Immediate.
2 Urgent.
3 Semi-urgent.
4 Delayed.

With all systems the success depends on the operator. Consequently the nurse's decision must be based on a sound knowledge and skill base. Despite this individuals will still differ in their interpretation of urgent, semi-urgent and delayed and this supports the need for a triage nurse to be in post for each duty period of the day. It also supports the introduction of a priority rating guide. The use of time attached to the various categories can also help individuals decide on the category:

1 Immediate – at once.
2 Urgent – within 15/30 minutes.
3 Semi-urgent – within 30/60 minutes.
4 Delay – within 60/90 minutes and beyond.

The use of a timing system must be practical and based on individual departments' waiting time. Therefore it needs to be organized locally.

Patient
{
Immediate   Priority 1
Urgent   Priority 2
Semi-urgent Priority 3
Delayed   Priority 4
}

Fig. 3/2   The four-category rating scale

Priority rating guide (Table 3/1)

The majority of patients can be placed in the correct category if a priority rating guide is created. The guide allows the nurse to use her experience and knowledge and with the discovery of key signs and symptoms the nurse can usually categorize quite effectively. The use of algorithms (Fig. 3/3) may also be useful for determining urgency rating and may help the nurse decide on the category with more accuracy.

Colour coding

The use of colour coding can have very beneficial effects when determining the urgency of need. When used in the disaster situation, the colour coding should be nationally agreed. Red – Priority One. Yellow – Urgent, Priority Two. Green – Delayed, Priority Three. The coloured labels assist with easy identification of priorities. Within the A & E department similar colour coding can aid the use of priority rating and provides an easy method of identifying those patients who require priority care.

Medical specialty triage (Fig. 3/4)

Another method of categorizing patients is by the apparent nature of their medical condition as well as the need for priority care. This system is underused in most UK A & E departments, primarily because the current system requires every patient to see the A & E Senior House Officer. As departments develop with nurse specialists (nurse practitioners) this method of triage may become more acceptable. Many patients would benefit from the decrease in medical intervention, e.g. only one doctor undertaking the p.v. examination of a lady suffering gynaecological problems, and many would benefit from referral more immediately to the specialist firm, e.g. cardiac patients direct to coronary care.

	Red – immediate	Yellow – urgent	Green – semi-urgent	Blue – delay
Limbs general	Pulseless limb Gross deformity Compound fracture	Swelling, deformity Pain ++	Some swelling, no deformity Pain +	Very little swelling, no deformity, vague pain
Ankle	Pulseless foot Gross deformity Compound fracture	Unable to weight bear Severe swelling Deformity	Weight bearing swelling	Old injury, weight bearing, very little swelling
Wrist	Pulseless hand Gross deformity Compound fracture	Swelling Deformity Pain ++	Some swelling Movement fair Not in severe pain	No obvious swelling Movement good Slight pain
Wounds	Uncontrolled bleeding Arterial damage Hypovolaemic shock probable	Bleeding pronounced Wound gaping (held by pressure bandage) Contaminated wound	Bleeding, but normal dressing will hold May require sutures	Small superficial wound Tiny scratches
Head injury	Unconscious Abnormal neuro-observations	H/O unconscious Drowsy Dizzy Vomiting	H/O some dizziness not k.o'd No vomiting	Looks well No dizziness or nausea Fully conscious and orientated
Eye	Damage to cornea or globe Burns to eye Sudden total loss of vision	VA Corneal FB observed	VA normal Red and sore eye	VA normal Eye very little redness
FB's	If causing further damage to vital organs Pain ++	Deeply imbedded Pain ++	Imbedded Pain, minimal	Superficial FB No pain or vague pain only
Epistaxis	Uncontrolled bleeding Hypovolaemic	Bleeding	Oozing +	Stopped for check
Burns and scalds	Above 10% surface area	Skin loss Pain +++	Blister/redness Pain +	Redness Pain minimal
Neck pain injury	History suggests cervical spine damage	Severe pain Difficulty with movement	Pain + Movement slightly restricted	Vague pain Movement – good

Table 3/1 Priority rating guide

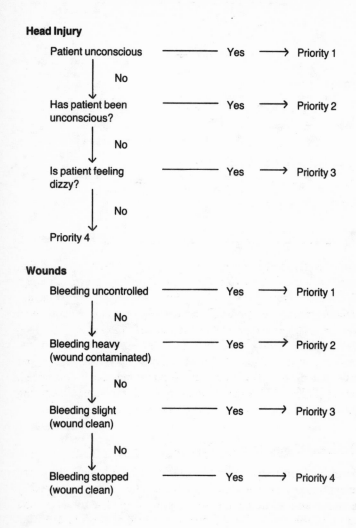

Fig. 3/3   Triage using algorithms

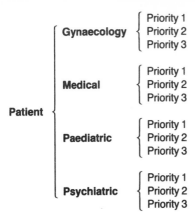

Fig. 3/4   Medical specialty triage

CREATING THE TRIAGE AREA

Having established a triage policy and given in-service training, suitable qualified staff will now be able to practise triage. Although in a disaster situation triage is very rapid and usually performed at the front entrance to the A & E department, on a day-to-day basis a more formal approach needs to be organized. A triage area needs to be established. This area should ideally allow triage of all patients. However, owing to the design of many departments this is not always practicable. Two types of triage setting can be discussed. One is the ideal. The other is what can be achieved in reality, taking into account the department's geography and financial restraint.

The ideal triage setting (Fig. 3/5)

The ultimate in triage setting is a purpose-built triage area at the one entrance to the department, where all patients can be triaged by the nurse and allocated the appropriate area of care. This area should afford good views of the waiting-room, provide a private examination cubicle and facilities for first aid care, and should have adequate hand-washing facilities. The area should have a patient locator board and be serviced with telephones, departmental intercom system, emergency phones and radio link with the ambulance service and police.

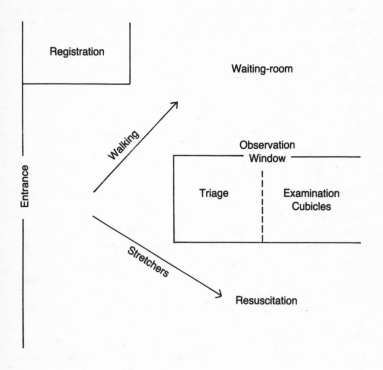

Fig. 3/5 The ideal triage setting

Sufficient trained nursing staff should be on duty to allow an identifiable nurse to staff the triage area throughout the 24 hour period. The nurse should be the first person to meet the patient, relatives and friends before registration takes place. The waiting-room is the triage nurse's 'Clinical Area' and must be treated as such.

Reality

The reality of setting up a triage system will often fall between currently having no system and the ideal. The first consideration is the reality of one nurse seeing all patients on arrival. Does your department have two entrances? Is it possible to achieve triage of both entrances by basing the triage point centrally? Because of the design, do you need to consider triage of the walking patients, separately from the stretcher patients? These question need to be considered carefully so the best setting for your triage area can be achieved. Many departments are designed in such a way that triage of all patients by one nurse at a triage point is impossible. It is necessary therefore to concentrate on two separate triage systems, one for the walking patient, the other for the stretcher patient.

Stretcher patients

This area of care does not cause a major problem. Most departments will work on a system of a senior nurse being in charge of the stretcher cubicles. This nurse should assess the patients in her area and prioritize them appropriately. Liaison with the triage nurse at the walk-in triage point will allow for continuity to be maintained between the two areas.

Setting up a walking patient triage area

The benefits of a formal triage system have already been discussed and therefore the setting up of a triage point to allow assessment and prioritization of all patients who walk into the department is essential.

Staffing levels will influence the setting up of the formal triage area. Do the present staffing levels in your department allow for a triage nurse to be identified? If staffing levels are a major problem, can an interim system be introduced while a bid for funding of a triage nurse is made? Always remember that triage can be effective without any major cost implications. The making of a good triage system is not the setting, but the commitment from the staff and the achievement of the goals of triage.

Location of the triage area should, if possible, be near the walk-in entrance and close to, or amalgamated with, the registration desk. The patient should be seen by the nurse first and then directed to the receptionist. It is preferable to have an area for private consultation if necessary, and the nurse should not simply sit at the reception desk. She will soon become a substitute clerk. If because of the geography of the department it is impossible to locate the triage point near the entrance, a desk should be placed in or near the waiting-room, or a specific triage area identified within the treatment cubicles and patients directed to this. If this method is used, it may be necessary for registration to take place first, so as not to create confusion with patients going back and forth.

Equipping the triage area

Ideally, all communications should come through the triage point. Phones and intercoms should be available. A patient location board should be used to maintain a clear picture of the current trolley availability.

Within the triage area the following should be available:

1 Dressings and bandages:
   Gauze.
   Strapping.
   Slings.
   Conforming bandages.
   Eye pads.
   Cervical collars.
2 Sphygmomanometer.
3 Stethoscope.
4 Pen torch.
5 Visual Acuity Charts.
6 Thermometer.
7 BM stix and colour code chart or machine.
8 Vomit bowls.
9 Ice packs or ice-making machine.
10 Documentation sheets/cards.

11 Local information – GPs, dentists.
12 Health education literature.

THE TRIAGE NURSE

Acting as the triage nurse can be very alien to the nurse during the first few weeks. Many nurses will feel uncomfortable with this extra responsibility and also the watchful eyes of the patients in the waiting-room. Senior accident and emergency nursing staff must be available to support and supervise the more junior nurses and the time each nurse spends at triage should be limited. The nurse should triage each patient according to the agreed policy and using the A & E model. The assessment must be documented and priority rating determined. Small, coloured stickers can be used to identify the priority category allocated.

EXPLANATION TO PATIENTS

It is essential to explain the triage system to all patients, especially those who will be sent to the waiting-room. Most people will usually accept a reasonable wait if the system of priority rating is explained. The triage nurse must indicate through the establishment of the partnership that patients in the waiting-room are her responsibility and the invitation should always be given to return if necessary to the triage area for re-assessment. The triage nurse should also plan re-assessments of the waiting-room patients so no patients are forgotten. When re-assessed, the patient's priority rating will often remain unchanged, but no rating is absolute and if appropriate, the nurse can change the priority according to the new problem. A system of seeing all patients, even those in the delayed category, as soon as possible should be employed. The use of time-scales between the immediate and urgent categories and a 3:1 ratio for the other two categories is one method. Working on the four-category system, the seriously injured are seen immediately. Those patients in the urgent category are seen within half an hour and then three semi-urgent patients are seen for every one delayed patient. This ensures that the semi-urgent patients are seen before the delayed patients, but that the delayed patient is not constantly left without medical care. This method allows care to be given in a logical priority order but ensures the patients in the delayed category are still seen in reasonable time.

Further advantages of triage

Once a triage system has been established a sense of order occurs. Patients feel more comfortable having been seen and assessed by a trained nurse and first aid care having been provided. All patients are seen in priority order and this reduces the waiting time of many patients who require the service of the department.

Determining the patient dependency for nursing care

One of the universal goals of the accident and emergency model is to achieve a level of independence in the patient. Before any nursing intervention can adequately be performed, the nurse must identify the degree of patient dependency. Is the patient totally dependent on the nurse, e.g. cardiac arrest, or does the patient require minimal nursing intervention, e.g. injury to the little finger? Many patients will have more than one factor that determines the dependency and thus the amount of nursing care required, e.g. a patient suffering an eye problem would not normally require a high level of nursing intervention. However, if that patient was blind in the uninjured eye, and was now suffering injury to his good eye, a high degree of nursing care may be required. Incontinence may not cause the patient to become totally dependent on the nurse, but loss of mobility plus incontinence would.

The use of a patient dependency rating scale (Table 3/2) helps the nurse determine the category of dependency the patient will occupy and thus the level of nursing care that needs to be provided. Such a scale can only be a guide, and the nurse must always use her knowledge and skill to determine the patient's dependency and thus the care required. The dependency rating scale uses the seven

Communication

Able to communicate through all senses/co-operative and relaxed	1
Impairment of senses/demanding/anxious/tearful	2
Inability to use senses/disruptive/distressed	3
Total loss of senses/hysterical/aggressive	4

Airway, breathing, circulation

Independent control of ABC	1
Impaired control of ABC	2
Severe impairment of ABC	3
Cardiac/Resp. Arrest	4

Mobility

Fully mobile	1
Partial loss of mobility	2
Cannot mobilize without aid	3
Total immobility	4

Environmental safety and health promotion

Shows/expresses cognition	1
Not fully able to understand	2
Unable to understand	3
Demonstrates danger to self	4

Personal hygiene

Shows ability to maintain own hygiene	1
Appears to require supervision	2
Unable to maintain personal hygiene without assistance	3
Total loss of independent self care	4

Eating, drinking, elimination

Normal control/intake	1
Partial loss of control/intake	2
Loss of control – urine/bowels/vomiting	3
Double incontinent/Hyperemesis	4

Score

6–7 Low dependency	4
7–11 Moderate dependency	3
12–20 Higher dependency	2
20–24 Total dependency	1

Table 3/2   Dependency rating

components of life. Each component has four levels of dependency rating from total independence to total dependence. When the score from all the components is added together the dependency rating of the individual can be determined. The use of a four-category nursing dependency system conveniently links with the four-category urgency rating scale, recommended earlier. The nursing dependency system is based on the patient's nursing, rather than medical needs. It identifies key nursing areas, such as pressure area care, mouth, eye and skin care, mobility, observation of vital signs, urine output, i.v. fluid input, limb positions, drainage from wounds and *in situ* drains. It also identifies care in relationship to human behavioural activity, such as disruptive and aggressive behaviour. The system can be identified as with the urgency rating scale with dependency numbers (Table 3/3).

Patient dependency 1 – total dependency
Patient requires one or more of the following:
1 Nurse presence at *all* times.
2 Frequent (15 min.) vital signs to be taken and recorded.
3 Constant airway attention.
4 Resuscitation.
5 Rapid I.V. fluids.
6 Frequent pressure area care/use of pressure area devices/lifting.
7 Frequent mouth care, elimination support.
8 Constant attention due to behavioural problems.

Patient dependency 2 – high dependency
Patient requires one or more of the following:
1 Constant observation from nursing staff.
2 Vital signs to be taken/recorded ½ hour/hourly.
3 Observation/intervention with airway care.
4 Frequent I.V. fluid administration.
5 Regular pressure area care/use of pressure area devices/lifting.
6 Assistance with urinal/bed pan.
7 Frequent attention due to behavioural problems.
8 Care and discussion due to bereavement.

Patient dependency 3 – Moderate dependency
Patient requires one or more of the following:
1 Nurse available in calling distance.
2 Vital signs 2/4 hourly.
3 I.V. fluids.
4 Pressure area care 4/6 hourly.
5 Assistance with toiletry/commode/walking to toilet.
6 Reassurance/psychological support.

Patient dependency 4 – low dependency
Patient requires one or more of the following:
1 Nurse available in department.
2 Vital signs once only.
3 First aid prior to waiting for medical care.
4 Reassurance.

Table 3/3 Dependency categories

1 *Patient dependency 1* – Patients requiring total nursing care due to poor physical condition, either acutely ill/injured, because of severe behavioural problems or due to being chronically ill or terminally ill. For convenience the acutely ill/injured patient, can be classified as patient dependency 1A and the chronically ill or terminally ill

patient classified as patient dependency 1B.

2 *Patient dependency 2* – Patients who require a high level of nursing intervention due to physical condition; the amount of nursing input to this patient is less than the dependency 1 patient.

3 *Patient dependency 3* – Patients who require moderate levels of nursing intervention and are encouraged to be independent.

4 *Patient dependency 4* – Patients who require minimal level of nursing intervention and are self-caring.

The patient dependency should be assessed at the same time as the priority for medical care is being determined (Table 3/4). An immediate priority rating for medical care will often also indicate a high degree of patient dependency, but this is not always the case. A terminally ill patient may well be totally dependent for nursing care, but have a low priority rating for medical attention.

Summary

Triage means to sort, pick, place in priority order. Using a triage system in the Accident and Emergency department creates an environment conducive to the provision of a high-quality service. Triage allows assessment of all patients to be conducted in a controlled manner and ensures patients are seen according to priority of condition not time of arrival. Various systems can be adopted; the four-category scale has been recommended because of its flexibility.

The triage area must be identified with due regard to the geography of the department.

Patient dependency for nursing care should be determined during the triage phase. Once this is done, the nurse has a complete picture of both the patient's medical priority and nursing needs.

Patient with head injury

Patient's condition	Priority rating	Nursing dependency	Patient's nursing needs
Unconscious	1	1	Nurse present Airway care
Abnormal neurology observation			Position on side P.A. relief 15 min neurological observations Total nursing support catheter
H/o unconsciousness Drowsy	2	2	Nurse observation ½ hourly neurology observation Vomit bowls
Dizzy Vomiting			Reassurance Mouth washes
Some dizziness No vomiting	3	3	Nurse available Neurological observations 2 hourly Explanation/reassurance
No dizziness Fully conscious	4	4	Initial triage One set of neurological observations
Looks well			Patient can wait in waiting-room

Table 3/4 Example of patient dependency (nursing) and priority rating for medical care, working together

PART TWO

The Process of Accident and Emergency Care

4 *Assessment*

The nursing assessment is the first and one of the most essential steps in the problem-orientated approach to care in the A & E department. Unlike the ward environment, the patient entering the A & E setting has not been seen by any other health care professional and therefore the nursing assessment will determine the problem, dependency, goal, priority status and the intervention required. There are a number of skills the nurse must acquire before she will be able to make an efficient assessment of any patient:

1 *Interviewing skills* – listening, reflecting, clarifying.
2 *Judgemental skills* – drawing clues and inferences from information.
3 *Observation skills* – sensitivity to non-verbal behaviour and interpersonal responses.

In addition to these skills, the nurse must have a framework to follow so no area of assessment is missed.

The assessment must be based on the seven components of life. This will ensure a smooth passage through the care process. Inadequate or incorrect nursing assessment can lead to inappropriate intervention which will not allow the patient to regain independence, health and quality of life, or loss of life. The assessment should be performed in two stages:

1 The general or first-stage assessment
2 The second or in-depth assessment.

The first-stage assessment will be carried out by the triage nurse and then a more detailed second-stage assessment will be carried out either by the triage nurse, or the primary nurse. The decision to carry out the second-stage assessment at triage or within the clinical treatment area, will depend on the patient's condition and the departmental activity.

The general assessment stage

This first stage of the assessment is normally carried out by the triage nurse and allows for an overall picture of the seven components of life to be obtained and the identification of those components that require a more in-depth, second-stage assessment. The general assessment will always commence with the assessment of the communication component, thereafter the sequential order will depend on the patient's overall condition.

The triage nurse needs to acquire details relating to personal data, name, age, address, etc. The nurse needs to discover the subjective information, e.g. what the patient knows, feels, what the patient tells you. The objective information is what the nurse knows, feels, and sees (examination). The nurse must analyse the information gained from both the subjective and objective information and then make a plan of action based on that analysis. This method of gaining the information required is termed the S.O.A.P. (Subjective Objective Analysis Plan) Nursing Assessment.

Many patients will assist the nurse in making a valid assessment. The patient who has a wrist injury will often launch straight into the whys and wherefores of the problem and without request will indicate the area of discomfort, thus providing the nurse with most of the details required. Other patients will not be able to provide such details and the nurse will need to probe deeper.

COMMUNICATION

1 Is the patient conscious or unconscious?
2 What is the purpose of the visit to A & E?
3 What is the chief complaint?
4 Is the injury primary or secondary?
5 What human behavioural signs and symptoms are exhibited.

6 Are any of the physiological senses affected?
7 Is the patient exhibiting signs and symptoms of pain?
8 Is the patient wearing any medic alert?
9 Does the patient suffer from any allergies?

AIRWAY, BREATHING, CIRCULATION

1 Is the patient breathing, ventilating adequately?
2 Is the patient's airway clear?
3 Is there a heart-beat?
4 What is the patient's skin colour?
5 Is the patient showing signs of shock?
6 Is the patient suffering from haemorrhage, burns or scalds?

MOBILITY

1 Has the patient come into the department walking, in a chair or on a stretcher?
2 Is the patient limping, having difficulty with walking?
3 Is the patient supporting a limb, are all limbs moving?
4 Has the patient difficulty with the neck?
5 Is the patient's gait normal?

EATING, DRINKING AND ELIMINATION

1 Is the patient vomiting?
2 Is the patient complaining of inability to pass urine?
3 Inability to open the bowels?
4 Has the patient got diarrhoea?
5 Is the patient large, thin, hydrated or dehydrated?

PERSONAL CARE

1 Is the patient dressed smartly, poorly, work related?
2 Is the skin clean, dirty or work related?
3 Does the patient have a body odour?
4 Is the hair tidy or unkempt?

5 Is the general appearance work related or due to inadequate personal care?

ENVIRONMENTAL SAFETY

1 Is the injury/condition due to inadequate work or home safety?
2 Is the A & E environment safe?
3 Is the correct amount and skill mix of staff present, e.g. is the surgeon available to the trauma patient?

HEALTH PROMOTION

1 Is the condition/injury due to poor self-care?
2 Is the condition/injury appropriately treated in A & E?
3 Is the patient suffering from a communicable disease?

Having performed the general assessment and identified the initial problems, the components now require further assessment. The Stage II specific assessment now takes place.

THE SPECIFIC (IN-DEPTH) STAGE

This second-stage assessment may be performed by the triage nurse or the primary nurse. One or more components will be present. The communication component always features in this stage. It provides the in-depth history and also allows the partnership to develop.

Communication

History
A detailed history is essential. The history can be obtained from the patient, relative, friends or other health care personnel, e.g. ambulance staff. If the patient is conscious, orientated and able to provide a full history, the nurse can obtain as much information as necessary. The nurse should not place words in the patient's mouth, but should ask open questions, e.g. 'Can you describe the pain?' rather than 'Is the pain sharp?' The history should include:

1 What is the exact nature of the complaint or injury (the chief complaint)?
2 When did the problem first occur and is there any previous relevant history relating to today's problem?
3 Has the patient taken any self-medication?
4 Any self-care advice?
5 Does the patient suffer from any allergies?
6 Is the patient immunized, e.g. tetanus covered?
7 Is the patient in pain?
8 Where is the pain?
9 Ask the patient to describe the pain. Is the pain associated with movement?
10 Is the pain referred, e.g. chest pain can be referred to the left arm? Bleeding from the spleen can irritate the diaphragm and referred pain will be felt in the left shoulder.
11 How long has the patient had the pain?
12 Has it become worse, easier, or remains the same?
13 Is the patient showing non-verbal signs of pain, e.g. facial expression, tears in the eyes, perspiration, etc?

Use of a pain scale can help assessment. Relatives and ambulance personnel can often provide other essential information relating to the mode of injury and the condition of the patient prior to arrival in A & E. If the patient was in a road accident the amount of damage to the vehicle, and the position of the patient, e.g. driver or passenger, can all help in the assessment of potential injury. The record sheet provided by the ambulance service should be referred to. This indicates what pre-hospital care has been given. Social history should be obtained where relevant. Has the patient any dependants? Does the injury/illness cause problems for the dependant? If a parent, has the patient left young children at home?

Assessing the conscious level

A patient who is conscious is able to respond to verbal stimuli. A patient who is unconscious will not respond to verbal stimuli and may or may not respond to pain stimuli. Assessment of the conscious state is best achieved using three parameters. The eyes, best verbal response and best motor response. A patient whose eyes open spontaneously, who is orientated to time and place and obeys commands, is what is often termed fully conscious. Various degrees of consciousness can occur, but use of such vague terms as semiconscious should be avoided. An accurate history from relatives or bystanders is essential if a patient has been unconscious. The exact length of time a patient was unconscious is essential. (If a patient was unconscious for more than 5 minutes following a head injury, the patient must be admitted for 24/48 hours observation, to exclude an intercranial bleed.) If the patient is unconscious on arrival in A & E, the time the patient became unconscious is required. The cause of the depressed conscious state is also essential. Is it due to trauma to the head? Or to the overdose or misuse of drugs or alcohol? Or did the conscious state deteriorate with no obvious cause? If the patient was found at the bottom of the stairs unconscious, was the unconscious state the cause of the fall? Or was the fall the reason for the unconsciousness? History will often help. If the patient shouted, he was conscious before the fall. If not he probably was unconscious beforehand. Also remember the empty medicine bottle does not always imply overdose. Check the date of dispensing and the daily dosage. It could be coincidence that the last tablet of the course was taken before the unconscious state occurred. When a detailed assessment of the conscious state is required the use of a coma-scale is necessary. The most widely used scale is the Glasgow Coma Scale. The scale consists of three sections:

1 *Eyes open* – Spontaneously, to speech, to pain, none.
2 *Best verbal response* – Orientated, confused, inappropriate word, incomprehensible sounds, none.
3 *Best motor response* – Obeys commands, localizes pain, flexion to pain, extension to pain, none.

When assessing the conscious state using the scale, the nurse must ask questions to which she knows the answer. It is pointless to ask the patient his name if you cannot confirm this with relatives or friends.

Human behavioural assessment

When talking to the patient and developing the partnership, the nurse will be able to assess the patient's behaviour. Is the patient relaxed? Cheerful? Quiet? Tense? Anxious? Aggressive? Agitated? Restless? Shouting or crying? Is the patient's mood suicidal? Are alcohol or drugs possibly affecting the behaviour? Is there a smell of alcohol? The patient's behaviour may be due to a sense of failure, especially if admitted because of an overdose or attempted suicide. Bereaved relatives will react in various ways and the nurse should be prepared for various ranges of distress. A patient's religious beliefs are important and will be reflected in behaviour and attitude.

Physiological senses

Assessment of the five senses may be required. Is the patient deaf? Does he have a hearing aid at home? Is this why communication is difficult? Is there any discharge or loss of fluid (CSF) from the ears? Has the patient lost the sense of smell? Assessment of the sense of touch is essential in any limb or spinal injury. Nerve damage or disease can create a loss of sensation. It may result in total loss of sensation or a feeling of pins and needles. Mouth injuries or dental problems can cause a loss of taste. Injury or infection to the eye is a very common problem seen in A & E. Infection of the conjunctiva causes a red, sore eye. Foreign bodies caught on the conjunctiva or cornea are also common conditions seen. Assessment of the eye must be performed following a detailed history of the problems. It is essential to know if the condition is due to trauma and if the injury was blunt or of a high velocity nature e.g. flying pieces of metal from a grinding wheel. The nurse must determine whether the patient wears glasses or uses contact lenses. Both eyes should be examined so a comparison can be made. Any complaints of blurred or double vision, of haloes around lights, flashing lights or floaters, should also be recorded. The visual acuity using Snelling's eye chart must be performed. This test not only gives the nurse an indication of the patient's vision, but also acts as a legal record of vision, prior to treatment.

Assessment of the eyes (Use a bright light)

   Lids – Any redness, encrustations, styes, cysts.

Conjunctiva – Any redness (conjunctivitis gives a classical redness peripherally, becoming less, nearer the cornea). Subconjunctival haemorrhage can often be seen. This can be due to trauma or occur spontaneously. Most spontaneous haemorrhaging is not significant; however, it could be due to hypertension or diabetes. Assessment of the blood pressure and blood sugar level will identify if this is the potential cause. Is there any discharge/tears/foreign bodies (subtarsal)?

Cornea – Is it clear or misty? Any injury to the cornea, any foreign body present? Use of fluorescein identifies any corneal abrasion?

Anterior chamber – Is the chamber present? Any foreign bodies, blood, pus. Is the pressure normal?

Pupil – Is it central, round? Does it react to direct light? Is the reaction painful? Painful reaction indicates a major eye problem, e.g. iritis, glaucoma.

Iris – Are there any wounds?

Lens – Is it present? Is there movement of the iris (iris wobble)? This indicates that the lens has either been removed (aphakic) or is dislocated due to trauma.

Globe – Is the globe intact? Are there any perforations of the globe?

Blowout fracture – Has the blow to the eye caused a fracture of the base of the orbit, with impaction of the inferior rectus muscle? This can be identified by the presence of diplopia on upward gaze and surgical emphysema around the cheek.

AIRWAY, BREATHING, CIRCULATION

The correct assessment of this component is essential to life.

Airway

The air passages can become partially or totally obstructed. The most common cause of the obstruction is the tongue, foreign bodies, vomit, injury or water when drowning. Assessment of the airway is essential, especially in the unconscious patient. A clear airway can be identified by the presence of normal ventilation of the lungs. No noise should come from the airway and expired air should be felt on the nurses' hand or cheek. Partial obstruction to the airway can be identified by noisy breathing. Various noises will be heard, depending on the cause. Partial obstruction due to a foreign body, or the tongue will often cause a snoring sound to be heard. Fluid in the air passages will cause a gurgling sound. Partial obstruction in the lower air passages, such as occurs in asthma, will cause a wheezing sound. Obstruction at the larynx can cause stridor. The respiratory pattern may be disturbed. If a patient is conscious and able to speak, partial obstruction may also be identified when the patient has difficulty in talking, or a hoarse voice. Total obstruction is identified by an absence of respiration. No sound from the airway but also no expired air can be felt on the hand or cheek. The nurse, when looking into the throat or nose, should use a bright light and if experienced in its use, a laryngoscope can be vital if medical aid is not immediately available. Soot, or red areas in the nose and mouth in the burn patient, indicate serious airway damage.

Breathing

When assessing the patients' ability to breathe adequately, the chest must be examined both from the front and back. Breathing can be impaired for a number of reasons:

1 An obstructed airway.
2 Insufficient oxygen in the inspired air.
3 Chest injury causing abnormal chest movement.
4 Pneumothorax, spontaneous or due to trauma.
5 Neurological damage to the respiratory centre and the nerves of respiration.

Pneumothorax can be a spontaneous event, or due to damage to the lung from rib fractures. An open wound to the chest will cause a pneumothorax and can be assessed by the noise of air being sucked through the wound on inspiration. Various medical problems of both the lungs and heart, will cause a change in respiratory physiology. Drugs can also cause respiratory depression. Chest movements should be observed carefully. Respiratory rate, rhythm and depth must be assessed. Under-ventilation, even with what appears to be normal respiratory movements, will soon lead to hypoxia. Hyperventilation can lead to a decrease in carbon-dioxide levels, causing an imbalance in the body chemistry and tetany results. The patient can show carpopedal spasm and hyperactivity of the facial nerve. Abnormal chest movements, especially paradoxical breathing, use of abdominal and accessory muscles, chain stoke breathing and gulping air like a goldfish, all indicates inadequate ventilation. Paradoxical breathing is due to a flail segment of chest wall, moving in the opposite direction to the rest of the chest wall. As the chest wall moves out, the flail segment sucks in, the reverse happening on expiration. Lung ventilation is grossly diminished. Cyanosis – especially of the ear-lobes, lips and fingernails – indicates poor oxygenation. A rather pink skin could also indicate poor oxygenation if related to carbon-monoxide poisoning. The patient's complaint of difficulty with breathing and the obvious shortness of breath will also aid the assessment. Persistent cough and haemoptysis suggests an underlying respiratory pathology. Air trapped in the tissues (surgical emphysema) or the chest wall can be felt when the chest is palpated. The surgical emphysema feels like bubbles popping under the skin. Respiratory arrest is identified by the patient being unconscious, absent respiratory movement and cyanosis of the skin. Clubbed fingers are a typical sign of a chronic respiratory problem.

Circulation

Assessment of the circulation may require the assessment of both the central and peripheral circulation, or just the peripheral circulation to one specific area of the body. Central circulation can be impaired, due to:

1　Pump failure (infarct), left ventricular failure
2　Loss of body fluid (external or internal haemorrhage, burns or scalds)
3　Central nervous system disease

Peripheral circulation will always be affected when central circulation is impaired. However, injury or obstruction of blood vessels in one specific area of the body may not have a dramatic affect on the circulation as a whole. The pulse and blood pressure indicate the general well-being of the circulation. The pulse should be assessed for its rate, rhythm and volume. Various abnormalities of the pulse indicate specific disorders. The blood pressure will rise and fall, usually in relationship with the pulse. However, in the recently injured patient, the blood pressure may remain a normal pressure despite obvious injury. This is due to good compensatory mechanisms of the body. Impairment of the central circulation is identified as shock. Shock is a sudden drop in blood pressure causing hypoxia to the tissues. The body's response provides classical signs and symptoms which can be assessed.

1 Pale skin.
2 Cold, damp skin.
3 Increase in respiration.
4 Confusion.
5 Increase pulse rate.
6 Urine output reduction.
7 The patient complains of thirst.

The blood pressure may not be recorded as low due to the compensatory mechanisms, but will fall dramatically if intervention is not immediately to hand. Cardiac conduction may be affected, especially with disorders of the heart. During the assessment stage an ECG and attachment to a cardiac monitor may be necessary. Cardiac arrhythmias may be present and the nurse should have a working knowledge of the more common ones, so that medical aid can be summoned without delay. Patients with heart conditions may complain of palpitations. Cardiac arrest is identified by the absence of the major pulses in the body (carotid or femoral). Because of the nature of cardiac arrest, respiratory arrest is also present and combined the signs are:

1 Unconsciousness
2 Lack of respiratory movement

3 Cynanosis
4 No major pulse.

Damage to the brain can have a dramatic effect on the cardio-vascular system, and increased pressure on the vaso motor centre and cardiac centre will lead to a decrease in the pulse rate and increase in the blood pressure.

Obstruction of blood vessels in the limbs will cause dramatic signs and symptoms. Venous obstruction will often cause a hot, red, painful, swollen limb. The most common venous obstruction is due to a deep vein thrombosis in the calf. The major risk to the patient from this condition is pulmonary embolism. The patient should therefore be assessed for any chest pain, especially if related to breathing. Arterial obstruction results in a white or cyanosed pain-ful, pulseless limb and is usually due to an embolism from other areas of the body.

Wounds to the skin will result in various degrees and types of blood loss. Simple wounds to the skin and subcutaneous tissue often bleed from damaged capillary beds. The blood oozes out and is dark in colour. Wounds affecting veins bleed more freely, and the blood is very dark and flows. Arterial bleeding results in a spurting of blood, which is often a much lighter colour. Assess the depth of the wound. Is there any foreign body present? Is there actual tissue loss? Other causes of bleeding can be due to erosion or damage to blood vessels, e.g. epistaxis, bleeding tooth sockets, bleeding from the ear following a head injury, etc. Bleeding under the skin surface results in bruising. When assessing a patient who has suffered a traumatic injury, bruising should be carefully assessed, especially if over vital organs, e.g. abdominal or chest injury. Some bruising will take on the pattern of the clothing or the cause of the injury, e.g. tyre marks on the body from the car wheel. Arterial vessel damage can result in poor circulation to other areas. The pulses distal to the injury can be absent.

Burns and scalds cause fluid loss and skin destruction. The assessment of the burn or scald should include estimating the area of tissue damage. The most common means of assessing such injury is with the use of the Wallace rule of nine, burn chart. The body surface is divided into percentage areas. The burn or scalded areas are added together and a total damage area estimated. In A & E the area of damage rather than depth is more crucial because the surface area assessment determines the fluid replacement.

A change in the metabolic activity of the body will affect the temperature, e.g. infective organisms. A rise in temperature often presents as a warm, flushed skin. The use of a clinical thermometer identifies the degree to which the temperature has risen. A drop in the body temperature (hypothermia) presents as cold, dry skin. The patient can be confused and dehydrated. Local reaction of the cardiovascular system to inflammation or obstruction/injury to blood vessels will affect the skin temperatures at local level.

MOBILITY

Assessment of the mobility component should be considered under two headings:

1 Mobility relating to one or more limbs.
2 General mobility of the body.

Mobility of limbs

Many patients present to the A & E Department complaining of injury to one or more limbs. The injury can be a sprained ankle or multiple fractures of several bones. Injury to the wrist, shoulder, ankle, clavicle or neck are very common. Other injuries often seen in the accident and emergency department are upper leg and arm injuries, injury to the pelvis and vertebral column. All the injuries create problems of mobility. During the assessment the nurse must establish the degree of mobility loss in the limbs or joints. Is there a deformity? Is the joint displaced? The patient should be asked to move the injured area but should never be forced if unable. The nurse should not actively move the limb or joint.

Tissue swelling will often be one of the major causes of immobility, and the nurse should assess the amount of swelling and/or deformity. Injury to tendons will cause varying degrees of immobility, as will fear, pain and nerve damage. Pain and immobility in a limb can be due to infection of the joint. The nurse should ensure that any problem relating to a joint is primary and not secondary to another problem, e.g. infection from a previous infective disorder elsewhere in or on the body. Injury to the spinal cord can cause varying degrees of immobility and weakness to the limbs. High cord damage can affect the movement of the arms as well as legs. Lower cord damage will only affect the legs. Male patients may show an erection.

General mobility of the body

Inflammatory or degenerative changes in the body will affect the mobility of many joints. The patient's mobility can be assessed using such criteria as:

1 Can the patient stand from a seated position?
2 Can the patient sit up in bed?
3 Is the patient able to walk unaided?
4 Does the patient fall to one particular side?
5 Can the patient walk with the aid of a frame or stick?

Assessment of the skin for pressure sores will also indicate if the patient has been immobile. Mobility can well affect the patient's ability to provide care to dependants. This area needs to be considered when assessing patients' specific components.

EATING, DRINKING, ELIMINATION

During the assessment stage of care, most patients are encouraged not to eat and drink. It is essential to establish with any patient suffering potential problems requiring an empty stomach, at what time they last ate or drank. When dealing with patients complaining of weight loss or dehydration, the patients' normal diet and fluid intake should be identified. Changes in digestion, swallowing or bowel movements should also be noted. The patient's weight may need to be recorded.

Inadequate intake of carbohydrates in the diabetic patient will cause a sudden drop in blood sugar level. Blood sugar levels can be assessed with the use of the BM or Dextro Stix. This should be routine in all patients with diminished levels of consciousness, patients with infected skin lesions and children complaining of abdominal pain. Elimination of body fluids can be observed and directly tested. Observation of the amount, colour, content and smell, often assists the nurse in identifying certain problems. Testing of urine, vomit or faeces, especially for blood, also aids the doctors' diagnosis, as do other routine tests of such fluids.

PERSONAL CARE

The initial assessment of a patient's personal care often comes from the condition of the clothes and shoes. The hair, hands and face also indicates if personal care is taking place. Stale smells of body perspiration suggest inadequate washing or bathing. Assessment of the body allows for total observation of all skin surfaces. Inspecting finger- and toenails also helps. Dirt under the nails and long, unkempt nails, suggest poor personal care. The nurse must find out if dirt on the skin and clothes is due to inadequate personal care, or is work-related. Dirt that is ground into the skin and dirty underwear usually indicate poor care. Clean body skin and clean underwear usually identify that although the rest of the body and clothes may be dirty and ragged, it is probably work-related. Lack of personal care is often related with a lack of mobility, inadequate facilities or some behavioural problem.

ENVIRONMENTAL SAFETY AND HEALTH PROMOTION

The nurse needs to understand the patient's work or home situation. The patient's head injury may be due to the individual not wearing a safety helmet. It may also be due to the company not supplying such protection. The guard on a saw machine may have been faulty or the patient may not have used it. The elderly patient may have fallen because of the loose stair carpet or it may be due to the lack of mobility and the bathroom being located upstairs. The lack of a handrail on the bath may be the cause of the fall from the bath. The patient who suffers from epilepsy and worked on a high building may be putting himself at risk. The cleaning fluid that the child has just ingested had been placed in a lemonade bottle and left at a low level.

Many patients have dependants. The nurse must assess the need for these dependants to be cared for. The environmental safety of the dependants is very important. It may require social services' intervention or ringing the child's school to inform the teacher of the parent's inability to collect the child.

Does the patient's behaviour/appearance suggest a lack of self-care? Nicotine-stained fingers, alcoholic smell on the breath, wearing inappropriate shoes when suffering from foot or ankle injury? Has the patient infected one eye from the other, because of lack of knowledge of the spread of infection? Has the patient come to the department with a communicable disease? Identification of some obvious lack of health promotion on the patient's behalf allows the nurse to plan what self-care areas need to be discussed.

Immediate assessment of the patient's past environmental safety and health promotion may not be appropriate, especially if a patient has serious injury or illness. However, patients that may be discharged from A & E will require self-care guidance, either relating to the current problem or to help prevent further problems in both these areas. It is essential, therefore, to assess these two components of life at an appropriate time during the A & E visit.

Examples of assessment, using the components of life

ASSESSMENT OF THE MULTIPLY INJURED PATIENT

The head to toe examination ensures no area of the body is neglected. General assessment moves immediately into specific assessment in such cases.

Communication – Is the patient conscious or unconscious?
Airway, breathing, circulation – Is there any obstruction? Is a major

pulse present? Observe the respiratory pattern, chest movements and respiratory rate. Are there any flail segments? Is there any open chest wound? Is there internal or external bleeding? Is the external bleeding from an artery, vein or capillary? Is there any tell-tale bruising or tattooing of the skin? Is the patient shocked? What is the pulse rate and blood pressure reading? Is the skin pale, cyanosed, a normal colour or rather pink? Is the skin temperature normal or abnormal? Is the abnormal colour or temperature, general or local? Are the peripheral pulses present?

Communication – What is the history? How was the injury sustained? Is the patient wearing a medic alert? Is the patient under the influence of alcohol or drugs? What is the level of the Glasgow Coma Scale? Are the pupils normal and reacting? Is there any sensory loss? Is there any discharge from ear or nose (CSF)? To what degree is the patient in pain? Where is the pain? How is the pain described? Is the pain referred? What is the patient's tetanus status? Has the patient any allergies?

Eating, drinking, elimination – When did the patient last eat and drink? Is the patient vomiting? Has the patient passed urine? Is there any blood in the urine? Is there any blood at the meatus? This suggests a ruptured urethra. Is the patient well nourished?

Mobility – Is there any loss of mobility in the limbs? Is there any obvious swelling, deformity? Is the neck or vertebral column injured? Is the pelvis intact? Is the weakness in the limbs due to limb or possible spinal damage? Has the male patient sustained an erection? This can occur with spinal injury.

Personal care – Is the patient's skin in good condition, conducive with good self-care? Are the patient's clothes, especially underclothes, socially clean?

Environmental safety and health promotion – Was a lack of environmental safety the cause of the accident? Was the injury work-related? Is the trauma response in the A & E department, adequate?

The use of the trauma score helps in the overall assessment of the patient. It consists of three parameters, the Coma Scale, Respiratory Rate and Arterial Blood Pressure.

ASSESSMENT OF PATIENT WITH A LIMB INJURY

Most patients attending accident and emergency following a limb injury will complain of a specific problem, e.g. an ankle injury, wrist injury, upper leg pain. The nurse must undertake the general first-stage assessment and then the specific second stage.

Example – ankle injury

General assessment

Communication – Patient is conscious; no injury to head. Chief complaint is limb injury (ankle). Patient complains of pain.

Airway, breathing, circulation – No obvious problem.

Mobility – Patient limps into department, difficulty in walking.

Eating, drinking elimination – Not relevant at this point.

Personal care – Patient in football clothes, fresh dirt on skin.

Environmental safety and health promotion – Football injury (if this ankle injury was due to the wearing of inappropriate shoes, e.g. no support to the ankle or unstable footwear (e.g. high heels). This would be noted and advice given regarding more appropriate footwear).

Initial problems identified – Ankle injury due to football accident.

Specific assessment

Communication – Full history of injury obtained. Did patient hear any noise from ankle when injured? Was he able to bear weight after injury? Does he suffer from any allergies? Is the pain mild, severe or unbearable? Does movement increase the pain? Is there any sensory loss in the foot?

Circulation – Is there a pulse distal to the injury? Is the skin colour of the foot normal, is the skin a normal temperature?

Mobility – Is the ankle swollen? Is there any deformity? What degree of mobility exists in the ankle? Is the lack of mobility probably due to pain, fear, nerve or tendon damage (e.g. Achilles tendon tear) bone or muscle damage, swelling or deformity? Can the patient bear weight?

Eating and drinking – When did the patient last eat and drink?

Once the specific assessment is complete problems and goals can be identified, appropriate priority rating set and intervention commenced.

ASSESSING PATIENTS SUFFERING CHEST PAINS

General assessment

Communication – Is the patient conscious? Chief complaint – can be central chest pain, though it can be described as either a vague ache or severe pressure on the chest wall. Ask the patient if he or she has had a recent cough or chest injury.

Airway, breathing, circulation – Does patient appear shocked? Is the pulse rate rapid and irregular/slow regular? Is the patient breathless? Is the skin cyanosed? Is the pain worse on inspiration?

Mobility – Normally the patient will come into the department on a stretcher and the patient will usually appear quite weak.

Eating, drinking, elimination – The patient may be vomiting clear fluid.

Personal care – Patients may be in night or work clothes.

Environmental safety and health promotion – Not relevant at this particular time.

Specific assessment

Communication – Detailed history. Pain – what was the duration of the pain before calling the ambulance? The patient should describe what the pain is like. Is it vice-like across the chest? Does the pain radiate the neck and left arm? Are there any allergies? Is there any past history, e.g. angina, previous infarction? Does the patient take glycerine trinitrate spray or tablets?

Airway, breathing, circulation – The patient may have difficulty with breathing. What is the respiratory rate? What is the pulse rate rhythm? What is the blood pressure recording? ECG will be performed. Patient will be attached to the monitor. Assessment of rhythm. Is there any cough? Any sputum production? Is there any pulmonary oedema? Is the skin colour both central and peripheral, normal, pale or cyanosed? What is the body temperature?

Eating, drinking and elimination – If the patient is vomiting, observe the amount of vomit and the colour.

Summary

Assessment of patients in the Accident and Emergency department is a skilled procedure, which should only be conducted by experienced Accident and Emergency nursing staff. It requires efficient interviewing, observational and judgemental skills on the part of the Accident and Emergency nurse.

The assessment should be conducted in two stages. The first or general assessment stage should occur immediately the patient arrives in the department. The second or specific stage should follow as soon as possible after the first.

Both the first- and second-stage assessments should be conducted by using the seven components of life, as identified in the model of nursing.

5   *Analysing and planning patient care*

Once the assessment phase of the process of care is complete, the nurse has a wealth of information that requires analysis, so the next stage in the process – planning – can be implemented.

Analysis – Identifying the Problems

From the information gained the nurse must make a synopsis and organize the information logically. She must critically examine each part of the information and identify that which is relevant and that which is not. The nurse will be in a position to withdraw one, or a number of problems that require intervention. These problems may be actual or potential, for example:

1 Julie is unable to stand without assistance (actual problem).
   Julie may fall if left alone (potential problem).
2 Mrs Smith has a deformity at the wrist due to trauma (actual).
   Mrs Smith may have impaired circulation to the hand (potential).
3 The wound on Steven's hand is deep and contaminated with earth (actual).
   The wound may be infected with tetanus bacillus (potential).
4 Mrs Crow is immobile (actual).
   Mrs Crow may develop pressure sores if not turned regularly (potential).

On many occasions the intervention from medical and nursing staff may create further problems, e.g. the administration of a general anaesthetic giving rise to potential airway problems.

Following the analysis of information and identification of the patient's problems the nurse is now in a position to plan her care.

Planning

Planning patient care within the A & E department, like assessment, should not be seen as a major paper exercise. Much of the planning will be reflected in the intervention the nurse makes to achieve a favourable outcome. It is an impossible exercise writing out a care plan for an unconscious patient, with airway obstruction, due to vomit, when the intervention must be immediate and based on the plan of action in the nurse's head. This plan will have been achieved through education and experience. Documentation as soon as possible of the intervention, e.g. suction and positioning of the patient, clearly reflects the plan made. The knowledge that the nurse uses in a nursing situation is at least as important as the action taken (Carnevali, 1973).

Many accident and emergency departments have attempted to use standard care plans to overcome the problem of preparing a written plan prior to the event. In my experience these have become nothing more than elaborate guidelines which are used in the same manner as policy and procedure books, currently in use. These books, plus reference material, on patient care within the A & E department, provide much of the theoretical knowledge the nurse requires regarding patient care.

Planning of patient care can be subdivided into:

1 Specific goals to meet the problems identified.
2 The priority in which the patient should receive medical care.
3 The patient's dependency.
4 The nursing intervention required.

SPECIFIC GOALS

These will interrelate with the universal goals already set, for example the second universal goal is the achievement of a level of independence in the patient appropriate to his condition. If the problem of airway obstruction due to fluid was present, the specific goal would be a clear airway. Once this specific goal had been achieved, then the universal goal would also be achieved. The patient would be able to breathe independently, appropriate to his condition.

Problem – Airway obstruction (makes independent breathing impossible).

Specific goal – A clear airway (independent breathing now possible).

Goals in the department should be practical and short term. It is useless creating goals that are impossible to achieve, e.g. a patient with a chronic respiratory disorder will not benefit if the goal is to achieve normal ventilation. However, a goal to achieve improved ventilation in this patient may be achievable.

THE PRIORITY IN WHICH THE PATIENT SHOULD RECEIVE MEDICAL AID

This will be determined using the priority rating guide, developed as a part of the triage system (see page 45). The priority may well be determined very quickly during the first-stage assessment or it may require the full two-stage assessment to be performed before a realistic priority rating can be achieved, for example:

A patient arrives in the A & E department suffering from an eye injury. Initial first-stage assessment would suggest from the patient's behaviour and relatives' concern, that a major eye injury has occurred. Without further in-depth assessment the patient could easily be placed in the immediate or urgent category for medical care. The second-stage assessment of the patient's eye however, could well reveal nothing more than a sub-tarsal foreign body and simple removal of this by the triage nurse provides the patient with immediate relief and therefore a delayed priority rating could be allocated.

In contrast a patient with a possible fractured elbow may present at the first-stage assessment, as a candidate for the semi-urgent category. However, on identifying the absence of a radial pulse in the limb an immediate priority rating would be allocated.

THE PATIENT'S DEPENDENCY

Like priority rating, the patient's dependency will be determined using the patient dependency guide which was also developed as part of the triage system (see page 57).

Once the goals, priority rating and dependency, have been determined the next stage of the process of care is the nursing intervention.

THE NURSING INTERVENTION

Nursing intervention will be based on the problems identified and the nursing care plan. Intervention may take place very rapidly, e.g. cardiac resuscitation or may result in health education, following analysis of all the data collected.

6 *Nursing intervention and evaluation*

Once the problems, priority rating, patient dependency and goals have been identified, nursing intervention can take place. Intervention in the A & E setting can be considered under three main care headings:

1 Intervention unrelated to medical care.
2 Intervention prior to medical care.
3 Intervention during and after medical care.

Four types of nursing intervention can be identified during any or all of the above periods of nursing care:

1 Preventative intervention.
2 Supportive intervention.
3 Informative intervention.
4 Active intervention.

Preventative intervention

To prevent a problem occurring. This intervention relates both to nurse and patient, e.g. to prevent infection the nurse must maintain an aseptic technique. The patient must refrain from touching the wound.

Supportive intervention

This intervention enables and assists the patient to achieve self-care, e.g. the nurse enables the patient to meet hygiene needs with assistance as required. This assistance may be from a Community Nursing Service that the A & E nurse has arranged.

Informative intervention

The giving of information, teaching the patient, e.g. the nurse will explain the need for the newly sutured wound to remain dry. The nurse will explain and teach the patient how to redress his own wound.

Active intervention

The action the nurse takes to ensure patient care. Often this intervention relates to technical aspects of care, e.g. maintaining a clear airway, the giving of drugs, etc.

It is clear when considering the four types of nursing intervention that most are used during any patient care activity, but depending on the particular problem and stage in the patient's condition, the four will be used in varying proportions.

Example: The diabetic patient who arrives in a hypoglycemic coma. Initially the patient requires nearly all active intervention, but once consciousness returns, the patient requires very little active intervention, but a great deal of supportive and informative information (Fig. 6/1). Intervention in any of the three main care areas depends on:

1 The personal skills of the nurse delivering the care.
2 The environment/manpower available.

PERSONAL SKILLS

The ability of nurses to carry out nursing care is based upon their experience, therapeutic and technical skills, that they have developed. Basic nursing skills, technical skills, interactive skills and observation skills are all necessary.

ENVIRONMENTAL/MANPOWER IMPLICATIONS

This involves the carrying out of the prescribed care either by the one who performed the prescribing or by another, so delegated (the

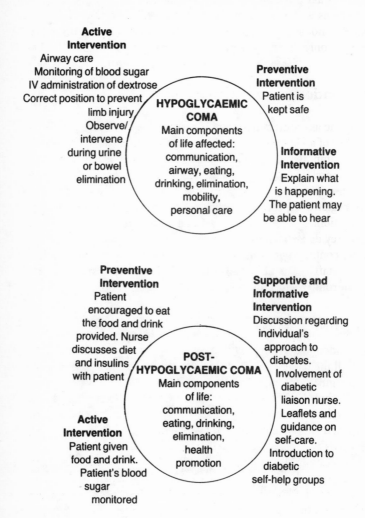

Active Intervention
Airway care
Monitoring of blood sugar
IV administration of dextrose
Correct position to prevent
limb injury
Observe/
intervene
during urine
or bowel
elimination

HYPOGLYCAEMIC COMA
Main components
of life affected:
communication,
airway, eating,
drinking, elimination,
mobility,
personal care

Preventive Intervention
Patient is
kept safe

Informative Intervention
Explain what
is happening.
The patient may
be able to hear

Preventive Intervention
Patient
encouraged to eat
the food and drink
provided. Nurse
discusses diet
and insulins
with patient

POST-HYPOGLYCAEMIC COMA
Main components
of life:
communication,
eating, drinking,
elimination,
health
promotion

Supportive and Informative Intervention
Discussion regarding
individual's
approach to
diabetes.
Involvement of
diabetic
liaison nurse.
Leaflets and
guidance on
self-care.
Introduction to
diabetic
self-help groups

Active Intervention
Patient given
food and drink.
Patient's blood
sugar
monitored

Fig. 6/1   Four categories of nursing intervention

primary or associate nurse). Delegated care involves effective communications and assurances that it has been accomplished. Intervention is not a paper exercise. It is the doing aspect of nursing which can only be observed in a practical setting.

Intervention unrelated to medical care

During the assessment period of care, the nurse will have identified a number of areas that do not require a direct medical input. One of the most important areas under this heading is the establishment of the partnership with the patient and relative. It also covers the prevention of pressure damage to skin. Other areas include personal hygiene care, bowel and bladder activity, patient's comfort and positioning in bed/trolley. Equipment within the accident and emergency department is also the responsibility of the nursing staff, and the continual presence of correctly functioning equipment and nursing staff with full knowledge of all equipment ensures that a safe environment for patient care is maintained.

COMMUNICATION

The accident and emergency department is an alien environment to nearly all the patients coming through the doors. Every department has its regular visitors, but most individuals will visit A & E perhaps once in their lifetime. During the assessment the nurse, patient and/or relatives will have developed a partnership and this will be maintained only if communication is continued between the two individuals and relatives, throughout the stay.

Identification of a primary nurse and associate nurses, working with the primary nurse, prevents an antagonistic situation developing between the nurses and patient and has a direct effect on the co-operation the nurse will receive from the patient. It is often the key to dealing with the human behavioural responses exhibited by the patient. B. Wright (1988) notes that much of the pain and distress in crisis is associated with a medical condition. The course of events of an illness or accident is closely linked to the eventual crisis. The specialist knowledge nurses have in linking the two is often vital to a patient's or relative's understanding of the whole situation.

The nurse, when dealing with the aggressive patient, can often prevent further confrontation, by talking to the individual in a non-authoritarian manner. Body language, especially facial expressions, can often make matters worse. Understanding the reason for the aggression will assist in diffusing the incident. Can the waiting time be reduced? Is the patient in pain? Is the patient influenced by drugs or alcohol?

Sudden death

Intervening in the sudden death situation is an area nurses will always find difficult. Informing and then staying with parents who have just lost their 10-year-old daughter in a road traffic accident is never easy. Emotional responses from the relatives will vary and the nurse must be prepared to deal with many different reactions. Withdrawal, denial, anger and crying, are just some of the emotions expressed. The nurse dealing with the relatives must be experienced in handling this situation. Many questions will need answers, both relating to the mode of death and what is to be done now. The nurse must be aware of all procedures regarding the coroner, the law, post-mortem, etc. Simple comments such as 'I understand' can be very unhelpful and may cause further anger and distress. Often it is appropriate not to say too much, but just to listen. The embarrassing periods of silence may be uncomfortable, but should be allowed. Relatives should be given time alone and never rushed out of the department.

ENVIRONMENTAL SAFETY

The accident and emergency department must be safe for the patient. Even Florence Nightingale (1860) stated that the hospital should do the patient no harm and it primarily falls to the nursing staff to achieve this aim.

Equipment

The equipment within the department must be appropriate for the type of care required. Beds and trolleys should be regularly maintained so that proper positioning of patients and transportation to other areas can be achieved.

Ideally the beds and trolleys should be of the variable height type. This aids patient care and prevents injury to the nursing staff. Oxygen cylinders must be full. It is pointless transferring a critically injured patient from A & E to ITU only to discover the cylinder becomes empty during the journey. Lifting aids should be considered, again, not only to aid patient care and comfort but also to prevent injury to nurses' backs.

Patients who are agitated or attempting to get off the trolley must be observed and trolley rails raised to prevent the patient falling. Very agitated patients or patients under the influence of drugs or alcohol are often best nursed with a mattress on the floor, thus preventing any risk of injury from a fall.

Electrical equipment, monitors, anaesthetic machines etc. must all have regular maintenance and a policy for dealing with such equipment when defective, must be available. All nursing staff should be familiar with all the equipment in the department and it must be the individual nurse's responsibility to ensure her continual up-date on equipment used infrequently.

Staffing

There should always be a sufficient number of trained A & E nursing staff to ensure good practice. Skill mix should allow for senior and junior nursing staff to be on duty throughout the 24-hour, 7-day week period. The staffing levels must reflect the knowledge that the patient may not be able to maintain safety in A & E if their medical condition puts them at risk: for example, loss of sight, inability to stand and walk, behavioural changes (e.g. confusion or drug-induced loss of control).

Infection control

Patients who are considered to have a communicable disease must have facilities to be nursed without the risk of cross-infection to other patients and staff. Appropriate areas and department policies should be produced so staff can practise safely and prevent any cross-infection.

Fire

Full and precise instructions for nurses on the procedure to adopt during a fire should be available. Nurses should attend fire lectures and practical demonstrations. Although all staff should be familiar with this area of intervention, many doctors are either in the hospital for a short period of time or are working locums, and therefore it falls to the nursing staff to take charge of such situations.

HEALTH PROMOTION

A department policy on health promotion should be established. Working with the health promotion team of the health authority can achieve great rewards. Health promotion literature and displays of current health interest allow the accident and emergency department and nursing staff to intervene in the health promotion of the local community. Many health problems seen in A & E can be prevented, if the patient is guided on self-care. This will range from correct footwear, personal care, diet, non-smoking, activity, etc.

PERSONAL CARE

Although in most departments it is the policy for all patients to be seen by the doctor, some patients have purely nursing and social needs. The individual who presents to the department with poor personal care may use the accident and emergency as his or her social welfare department. Although nursing staff should not encourage such a policy, it is inevitable that with the department open 24 hours per day, this type of care or need will present.

Many of the patients with personal care deficits will either be of no fixed abode or will have been living locally, but becoming unable to maintain personal care. It would be wrong, on a regular basis, to attempt to fill this gap in society, by nursing staff in A & E taking on the washing and reclothing of such individuals. However, it may be appropriate on some occasions to provide such care, prior to social services intervention.

The patient who, because of the lack of mobility or some other condition, cannot maintain personal care, must have this care provided by nursing staff. The elderly person being returned to the community should not be allowed to return in the same ill-kept condition that was present on arrival. Change of clothing should be either kept in accident and emergency or obtained from the care of the elderly unit. A good wash with hair and nail attention should be provided. Community nursing and social services should be contacted to prevent a return visit.

MOBILITY

Many patients, due to their illness or injury, have lack of mobility and therefore are at risk of developing pressure sores. This risk will be increased owing to other life components being imbalanced. The patient, depending on the condition, will probably be nil by mouth. Lack of personal care of skin may already be present. Age, weight, continence, type of illness or trauma will all have a bearing on the risk of developing pressure sores.

Always ensure that patients are not left lying on foreign material, especially following a road traffic accident. Many fragments of glass, metal or dirt will be under the patient when they are admitted to the department. If these are not removed at an early stage, these can cause local pressure sores. The same can occur owing to pressure from splints, cervical collars and other devices used to stabilize the patient's skeletal system. Spinal injured patients are at great risk from developing pressure sores and these can occur anywhere on the body, in a very short period of time. The hard trolley mattresses and the length of time some patients remain in A & E require strict nursing attention to pressure area care.

Unfortunately, because of the acute injury that many patients have suffered, it is not always appropriate to lift and move them constantly.

The elderly person suffering a fractured neck or femur does not take kindly to movement until in the ward environment, with counter-balanced traction applied. Therefore, much of the prevention in A & E is achieved with use of pressure-relieving devices and obviously, where able, turning the patient to relieve the pressure.

The use of sheepskin on accident and emergency trolleys and ankle sheepskin bootees help. Ankles should be lifted regularly and slight repositioning achieved. The use of pressure relieving mattresses on beds and trolleys will also help prevent pressure and many patients comment on the comfort achieved.

One of the most effective pressure area care systems is for the patient to spend the shortest possible time on the trolley in accident and emergency. This relies on the goodwill of the medical staff for speedy admission to the wards.

Intervention, prior to medical care

Having completed the patient assessment and organized both the priority rating and patient dependency, during triage, the triage and primary nurse will need to provide pre-medical nursing intervention. This intervention may be of the life-saving nature, such as cardiopulmonary resuscitation or as simple as placing a first-aid dressing onto a small laceration. The degree of intervention will depend on local policy and procedure.

Communication

PHYSIOLOGICAL SENSES

One of the most common interventions nurses will deal with, prior to the patient receiving medical care, relates to the eye. Many patients owing to their work or social activity, either suffer with foreign body in the eye, or from a chemical solution entering the eye. Chemical solutions should immediately be irrigated, either with tap water or normal saline. Use of buffer solution can be effective but may also create further chemical reaction. 200 ml of solution should be the absolute minimum used when irrigating eyes affected by chemicals, and often much more will be required. Once irrigation has taken place, medical care can be instituted. A sub-tarsal foreign body is easily removed by the nurse following assessment and reduces the risk of damage to the cornea. It is unacceptable practice to allow a patient to sit in the waiting-room following nursing assessment, with a sub-tarsal foreign body not removed.

Removal is simply achieved by everting the upper eye-lid and lifting the foreign body with the use of a cotton bud.

Airway, breathing and circulation

Airway obstruction can be due to the tongue or foreign material in the air passages. If obstruction has been identified then immediate intervention must take place:

1 The jaw must be lifted forward, thus allowing the tongue to be pulled from the airway.
2 Suction should be used to remove any foreign material.
3 A guedel airway should be inserted.
4 Ideally, the patient should be placed in the recovery position, but some injuries may prevent this and expert maintainance of the airway must be provided without exception.

BREATHING

The most common intervention nurses provide, prior to medical care, is oxygen administration and positive pressure ventilation. Many patients will present with breathing difficulties but a clear airway is noted. Oxygen administration is vital in such circumstances and should be administered immediately after assessment. The oxygen concentration to be administered must be determined.

This is either a low concentration for patients suffering chronic, obstructive airway disease or a high concentration for all acute conditions, especially when related to trauma.

Positive pressure ventilation should be provided to all patients in respiratory arrest. If the nurse is in a situation where no equipment is available (though this should not occur in A & E) mouth to mouth ventilation must be provided. Use of a resuscitation bag with oxygen is the method of choice. Another area of intervention, specifically related to breathing, is the immediate covering of open chest wounds. The nurse should use an airtight dressing over the wound to prevent further air entry into the chest cavity. This should be removed immediately if further respiratory distress occurs. Positioning of the patient in a semi-reclined position and to the injured side, will also aid ventilation in patients with paradoxical breathing. All patients with breathing difficulties benefit from sitting up in the bed and the nurse must adjust the pillows accordingly.

Reassurance from the nurse helps in reducing the patients' anxiety and hence respiratory difficulty. It is often the case that a patient with respiratory distress, having been positioned in a semi-recumbent or upright position, given oxygen and provided with the reassurance from a trained nurse, will improve prior to medical care.

CIRCULATION

Patients suffering from acute cardiac conditions need to be made comfortable in a semi-recumbent position as soon as possible. Oxygen administration and reassurance will aid in the reduction of stress being placed on the myocardium. If cardiac arrest occurs the nurse must immediately commence cardiac resuscitation and if the nurse is able, electrical defibrillation of the fatal arrhythmia should be initiated.

Bleeding

Any external wound should be covered with a temporary dressing to prevent further haemorrhage and infection. Burns and scalds should be cooled with tap water or normal saline. Temporary dressings of Cling-film should be applied, if it is appropriate or necessary for the patient to wait before being treated by the doctor. Patients suffering from shock due to severe haemorrhage, burns or scalds, should be placed on a trolley, flat. Oxygen administration and immediate medical aid should be summoned. If able the nurse should commence IV fluid administration.

Mobility

Patients suffering injury to one specific limb will often require nursing intervention, prior to medical care. Acute, swollen limbs due to possible sprains and strains require ice-packs to be applied and elevation to be achieved. Arm injuries are best supported in a sling and legs either elevated with the use of a leg support on a wheelchair, or by putting the patient on a trolley.

Splints should be applied to potential fractured limbs. Lower leg fractures are well supported using a box splint and upper leg fractures require the use of either a Thomas splint with fixed skin traction or the use of other traction splints, such as the Donway traction splint. The potentially spinal injured patient should be kept still and any necessary turning achieved by the use of the Log roll. Cervical collars should be placed on all potential neck-injured patients, but should not lead the nurse into a false belief that the neck is now immobile.

Eating, drinking, elimination

Patients must be encouraged not to eat and drink if they are assessed as suffering any condition where activity of the gastro-intestinal tract is not desirable. Patients who are vomiting should be offered vomit bowls, reassurance and mouth washes, as necessary. Patients who are complaining of retention of urine should be allocated a single cubicle and either a urinal or bedpan. Use of running water does help on occasions. Preparation of a catheterization trolley is prudent.

Personal care

Patients who require washing/showering and the issue of a clean examination gown, should have this done before medical intervention, where appropriate. Patients who, for whatever reason, have been unable to provide self-care, should not be left in a poor personal care condition any longer than necessary. Depending on the circumstances and medical presence, it may be desirable to allow the doctor a brief view before nursing care takes place, especially if follow-up and support care of the patient may be in dispute. Any patients who have been involved in any crime, even if they are the innocent party, should not have their skin washed or clothing removed, without thought for potential forensic evidence. Clothing should be placed in separate bags. Any foreign bodies from hair, wounds, etc. should be kept in specimen pots. Marks on skin should not be washed off, in case photographic evidence is needed.

Environmental safety and health promotion

This major area of patient care can well begin during the triage period. Many patients will have sustained injury or illness due to lack of environmental safety or health promotion. The nurse is in an ideal position to discuss these issues.

The child who has drunk from a bottle marked Lemonade, only to find dad has decanted Turps; the man who does not wear the mask provided and now is suffering from arc eyes; the carpenter who does not use the saw-guard and has cut his hand – all these patients can be advised on environmental safety issues.

Some patients may be inappropriately using the A & E department. If local policy allows, the correct health care facility can be recommended. Advice on the use of flat shoes when suffering from an ankle injury or not touching the infected eye and using individual towels when suffering from conjunctivitus, are all areas that can be explained to patients, thus promoting environmental safety and health care. Patients who, following assessment, are considered to be possibly suffering from a communicable disease, should be isolated and barrier nursing, if necessary, implemented.

Intervention during and after medical care

Nursing intervention during and after medical care will obviously depend on the particular problem. However, nurses must be prepared to assist medical staff as necessary and act as the patient's advocate during all medical intervention.

The partnership that should have been developed between the patient and nurse should not be broken, and the patient should identify the nurse as the link during the whole process of the A & E visit. During medical intervention it will normally fall to the nurse to explain what is happening and when. Many minor injuries are treated totally by the nursing staff, following medical assessment. Burns will be dressed. Sprained ankles strapped. What must be different between the nursing care and medical care, however, is what happens after the treatment has been given. The sprained ankle is a part of an individual who has now got to live for 10–14 days with a deficit of the mobility component of life. The nurse must therefore intervene, giving consideration to all the other components of life so that the individual can self-care, even with this deficit. This may require in some cases the intervention of relatives, social services or even temporary housing. It may require the issuing of walking aids and instruction on their use. Self-care advice on discharge can be given verbally and also in a written format. A number of departments have self-care advice slips, e.g. 'Care of your limb in plaster of Paris', 'Care following a head injury'. More specific intervention can be considered under the components of life.

COMMUNICATION

The unconscious patient – These patients must be positioned ideally on their side. The major care is of the airway. Always talk to the unconscious patient. Hearing may still be present.

The psychiatric patient – A patient suffering from a psychiatric disorder may require admission. Ideally after medical intervention, the patient will be admitted voluntarily. If the patient refuses voluntary admission, then it may be necessary to admit the patient under the Mental Health Act. The nurse will need to ensure all parties are clear as to which section the patient is being placed under. The nurse must ensure the appropriate forms are signed and that the patient is kept in a safe environment until taken to the ward.

Physical senses – corneal foreign body – Patients having suffered a corneal foreign body will have had it removed by the doctor. The nursing staff usually continue the care once this has been achieved. The application of the ointment and the eye-pad must be done with care. Ointment should be placed into the lower fornix of the eyelid. One eye-pad should be folded in half and placed over the closed lid. The second pad should be placed over the first and strapped down firmly. The pad should be left for 24 hours and the patient advised to return. The patient should be advised not to drive and not to touch the pad or the eye.

AIRWAY, BREATHING, CIRCULATION

Cardiac arrest

The nurse is a member of the resuscitation team. It is vital not only to carry out cardio-pulmonary resuscitation, but also to prepare the drugs required to stabilize the fatal arrhythmias. On discovering a cardiac arrest, the following intervention should take place:

1 Assess that cardiac arrest is present.
2 Summon help.
3 Place patient on firm surface.
4 Establish a clear airway.
5 Inflate the lungs – two slow inflations.
6 Check carotid pulse.
7 Commence cardiac massage – 15 compressions.
8 Inflate the lungs – two slow inflations.

9 Continue 15 compressions to two inflations.
10 Once help arrives, use a ratio of five compressions to one inflation.

Preparation of equipment should be considered in four stages:

1 Airway and breathing – equipment for intubation.
2 Cardiac activity – monitor and defibrillator.
3 Promotion of cardiac activity – IV drugs, e.g. atropine, lignocaine, adrenalin.
4 Access to circulation – Cannula.

Breathing

Intrathoracic damage can lead to air or blood collecting in the chest cavity. The nurse must be prepared to act quickly in support of the medical staff, especially if the air is under tension. The preparation and care of the tray for thoracic drainage must be performed. The thoracic catheter must be sufficiently large to allow good drainage. This catheter will be connected to an underwater seal drain that must be prepared by the nurse in response to the situation. Once in place the nurse must monitor the drain and ensure the 'swing' is present (swing is the movement of water up and down the tube leading to the patient and indicates air is being expelled from the chest cavity).

MOBILITY

Nurses will often assist medical staff in the reduction of patients' fractures. Apart from the care the patient requires due to the general anaesthetic, nurses will often apply counter-traction to the limb, while the doctor manipulates the fracture site. Application of plaster of Paris is performed by some nurses.

EATING, DRINKING, ELIMINATION

Following medical examination, many patients if in acute retention, will be catheterized by the nurse. Patients suffering constipation will have been prescribed an enema or suppositories. These will be given by the nursing staff, and the necessary care following the action will also require nursing intervention.

Patients who have taken an overdose of drugs will require either a stomach lavage or the administration of ipecacuanha syrup. Both will be delegated to the nurse.

Evaluation

Evaluation is basically a judgement of work – an appraisal of value (Suchman, 1976). It is the cornerstone to patient care. Unless evaluation takes place, goal setting and intervention is rather pointless. Evaluation must take place after any intervention. By evaluating the nurse can see if the care given achieved the goal set. Evaluation can be carried out by:

1 The nurse evaluating her own function.
2 Peer evaluation.
3 Management evaluation.
4 Patient evaluation.

COMMUNICATION

1 Has the partnership been established, if not why?
2 Has the unconscious patient regained consciousness?
3 Has the aggressive patient settled?
4 Is Mr Brown in cubicle two less anxious due to your intervention?
5 Have the relatives of the BID gone home with all the necessary information?
6 Has the patient with the foreign body in eye been seen and treated by the doctor?
7 Has the history been documented?

AIRWAY, BREATHING, CIRCULATION

1 Is the airway patent?
2 Did the suction and position create a clear airway?
3 Is the underwater seal draining well?
4 Is the oxygen administration improving the patient's colour?
5 Has the position of the patient helped the breathing?
6 Did the nebulizer relieve the bronchial spasm?
7 Has the pressure dressing prevented further blood loss?
8 Has the heart restarted, following cardio-pulmonary resuscitation?
9 Have the pulse and blood pressure improved?

MOBILITY

1 Can the elderly lady walk, now you have given her a stick?
2 Why did the patient fall when given crutches?
3 Has the Tubigrip bandage retained its position on the patient's knee?
4 Why did the patient develop pressure sores on her left heel?
5 Why does the patient keep slipping down the bed?

EATING, DRINKING, ELIMINATION

1 Has the stomach wash-out removed all the tablets?
2 Is the urine draining well through the catheter?
3 Did the diabetic patient receive the correct level of carbohydrates in his meal?
4 Has the patient stopped vomiting since the anti-emetic was given?

PERSONAL CARE

1 Is the patient's skin clean after the learner nurse washed the patient?
2 Does the patient appreciate the need to change his clothing regularly?

ENVIRONMENTAL SAFETY AND HEALTH PROMOTION

1 Why did the lady infect her other eye?
2 The elderly lady has not fallen in her bath since the handrail was fitted.
3 No children from that home have come again, having drunk turps.
4 That young lad still comes suffering from arc eyes.
5 No one comes to the department now who should go to the GP.

Evaluation shows if you have achieved your goal. Remember – it may not be your intervention that was wrong, if the goal is not achieved. It may be that you set the goal too high.

Summary

Intervention is the actual 'doing' stage of patient care. It is the time when all the assessment and planning is reflected in the care provided. Intervention can be carried out by the nurse who has planned the care, or the care may be delegated to another nurse. Care will vary in content depending on the identified problems. Some intervention will be of an active type, some a preventative and informative type, and other intervention can be supportive in nature.

Within the Accident and Emergency setting, three main care headings can be identified: (1) intervention unrelated to medical care, (2) intervention prior to medical care and (3) intervention during and after medical care. All intervention, irrespective of the category, will be provided using the seven components of life as the headings of care.

Evaluation is essential for judging the result of your intervention. The evaluation identifies whether the goals have been achieved. It allows, if necessary, a re-analysis of the problems and the re-establishment of goals.

7 Documentation

The key to good documentation in the accident and emergency department must be simplicity. The most simple way of obtaining a nursing record is to use either a plain sheet of paper or a blank accident and emergency record card. The use of such records allows the nurse to record the assessment, plan, intervention and evaluation, based on the nursing model in a totally individualized way.

The major problems, however, with using a blank sheet of paper or A & E card are:

1 All nurses must record in the same manner following the components of life.
2 The time spent on writing is prohibitive.
3 Less experienced nurses have no guide to follow.

In accepting these problems, some form of pre-printed document-ation needs to be developed and made available in the department, so all stages of care can be recorded. Various methods of docu-menting A & E nursing care have been attempted throughout the world. This documentation ranges from a simple list of activities which only records the assessment (Fig. 7/1) through to a full-care plan system. The majority of more detailed, pre-printed record sheets, currently available, allow documentation of the assessment stage of care and then revert to the plain sheets for ongoing intervention and evaluation (Fig. 7/2). Standard care plans have been developed by the RNA of British Columbia. These plans identify the anticipated problems, patient outcome criteria and standards, deadlines and nursing process standards (Fig. 7/3). The appropriate care plan should be identified following the patient assessment. A slight variation of this standard care system has been advocated by Walsh (1985).

Systems used within my own A & E unit, until quite recently, have allowed the nurse to record the various stages independently, but at the same time have given some general guidance (Fig 7/4). Although these documents have proved reasonably successful, they have again taken time to complete and consequently the full record of the assessment, intervention and evaluation, has not always been achieved.

They were impractical for use with patients suffering minor injuries where the turnover was very rapid.

Designing a document for use with all patients in accident and emergency

Many patients attending the accident and emergency department have similar problems. Most patients arrive complaining of a

	Assessment	Action
General appearance. Distress. Pain.		
Breathing.		
Circulation.		
Body temperature.		
Communication.		
Hygiene. Skin condition. Wounds. Swelling.		
Nutrition.		
Elimination and excretion.		
Mobility.		
Social.		
Assessment by:		Time:

✔ Indicates no apparent or relevant problem.

Fig. 7/1   Nursing assessment

Admission and/or Initial Patient/Family Assessment

Date		Time		Admitted from		via	
T.	P.		R.	B/P La.	Ht.		Wt.
Reason for hospitalization or chief complaint							
Duration of this problem							
Other illnesses							
Previous experience with hospitalization							
Observation of patient's condition							
Mental/emotional status							
Allergies							
Medications							
Prostheses							
Patterns							
Hygiene							
Rest/sleep							
Meals/diet							
Activity status							
Elimination – Bowel:							
Bladder:							
Menstrual history – LMP							
Health practices							
Life style							
Typical day profile							
Informant:							

The admission and/or the initial assessment is to be done by the R.N. within eight hours after admission.

Form # 1372   Cat. No. 4551   (10-76)

(SEE REVERSE SIDE)

R. N. Signature

Fig. 7/2   Nursing data base

				Emergency Unit
This standard care plan is intended for adaptation and ratification by each agency before being used.		Agency		
		Standard Care Plan	Cardio-Pulmonary Emergencies – Admission	ADDRESSOGRAPH STAMP
		Patient Population	Adult, any age or sex	
Date	Anticipated Problem	Patient Outcome Criteria and Standards	Deadlines	Nursing Process Standards
	1. Chest pain due to myocardial ischemia.	1. Experiences relief of chest pain. Scale # 1 Pain 1. Pain absent. 2. Pain lessened but not relieved by intervention. 3. Pain remains or increases despite intervention.	15 minutes post administration of I.V. morphine.	1. Complete standard nursing assessment. 2. Obtain data to chief complaint: 2:1 Chest pain 2:2 Edema – peripheral — dependent 2:3 Neck vein distention 2:4 Bilateral B.P. 2:5 Apical radial pulse 2:6 Chest sounds 2:7 Cough 2:8 Sputum – colour — consistency — amount 2:9 Urinary output.
	2. Respirator distress due to pulmonary edema.	2. Experiences relief of respiratory distress. Scale # 1 Respiratory distress 1. States he is breathing more easily. 2. Distress continues but less. 3. Distress continues.	1 hour after intervention.	3. Complete standard nursing intervention.
	3. Arrhythmia due to infarction.	3. Experiences relief of symptoms related to arrhythmia. Scale # 1 Rhythm 1. Normal sinus rhythm. 2. Arrhythmia controlled with intervention. 3. Uncontrolled arrhythmia.	Individual consideration.	4. Administer O$_2$ by mask @ ___ 5. Position semi-fowlers. 6. Monitor and record vital signs on flow sheets q ½ h. 7. Cardiac monitor.
	4. Nausea due to infarction and/or drugs.	4. Experiences relief of nausea. Scale # 1 Nausea 1. No further nausea. 2. Nausea continues but no vomiting. 3. Nausea and vomiting continues.	Responds within 1 hour of intervention.	8. Administer medications as ordered. 9. Initiate diagnostic procedures as ordered.
	5. Anxiety due to fear of pain.	5. Experiences relief of anxiety. Scale # 1 Anxiety 1. States he feels more relaxed. 2. Appears more relaxed with support. 3. Continues to express fears.	Depends on severity.	10. Record intake and output q ___. 11. Provide reassurance and explanation to patient and relatives.

© The Registered Nurses' Association of British Columbia, 1977

Fig. 7/3   Standard care plan form (design adapted with permission of Medicus Systems Corporation)

NURSING ASSESSMENT/RECORD ACCIDENT DEPARTMENT

ALLERGIES		ADMITTING NURSE	
Social Situation	Tick	Main Complaint	P
1) Lives with husband wife family			R
			T
2) Dependents yes no			B/P
3) Lives alone			
Community Services		History from Amb. & Patient	
Already provided: Nurse Social Services Meals on Wheels Home Help			
Housing		Treatment on route to Hospital	
House Flat Bungalow Warden Control Part Three Stairs			
Heating – Type Bath/Toilet Facilities		Nursing Assessment/Records & Drugs given including patient's requests, i.e. pets, security of house, etc.	Sig.
Discharge – Arranged TTA's EC 10 Follow up Ambulance Home To Clinic Social Services Nurse Meals on Wheels Home Help Someone at home on return			
Relatives Tick			
Present Gone home Informed Not known			
Telephone Number to contact while in Department			

Fig. 7/4   Nursing assessment record

particular medical or traumatic condition. Others have social, environmental safety and health promotional needs that must be addressed. When designing the nursing record for A & E, the first consideration is, should the record sheet be independent of the A & E card, or integrated? It was decided that an integrated nursing/medical document was the most sensible.

The next decision was how to achieve a pre-printed nursing assessment/intervention/evaluation record, while at the same time leaving room for medical documentation and not creating a set of notes that would be totally inappropriate when only a few lines is necessary to achieve total documentation.

The next problem relates to content. It is quite impossible to cover all types of problems the patient may present with on one pre-printed card. The decision was made therefore to use a system adopted from standard care plans and create several cards, identified by the presenting chief complaint (problem). Reassessment/add-on cards can also be available. The triage or primary nurse would make a first-stage, non-written assessment of the patient, identify the chief complaint and then choose the appropriate card. Use of add-on cards would allow patients with several problems to have adequate documentation. To allow the nurses rather than the reception desk to choose the correct card, triage can be carried out prior to registration or the documentation of patients' personal details can be taken at the reception desk and documented on a stick-on label. This stick-on label with the patient's details can be affixed to the card chosen by the nurse.

Future development of this system onto a complete computerized A & E patient quality care system is under discussion. It is hoped that patients once recorded at the registration desk and entered into the computer system, will be triaged, care plans provided and discharge self-care documentation achieved without the need for anyone to record their personal details more than once.

THE A & E CARD

The card consists of five sections. The inside of the card contains a pocket, and when the card is folded it creates a card measuring 15×20mm. When fully open the card measures 30×40mm. Section one consists primarily of the patient's personal details, triage status and brief history (Fig. 7/5). Section two consists of the nursing assessment section (Fig. 7/6). The assessment section of the document must allow for a detailed record to be obtained, yet also provide the nurse with ease of use. The decision was made to identify the key areas for assessment based on the chief complaint and allow a YES/NO tick system to be operated, thus cutting down on the need for lengthy note writing. The components for assessment are laid out in priority order and allow for both subjective and objective assessment.

**Basildon & Thurrock District Accident & Emergency Services.
Hospital**

Surname   Title   Chief Complaint

Allergies
Tetanus Status
Forenames   Priority   Dependency

Address   Triage Nurse/Primary Nurse

Time seen by Nurse

Planned reassessment every
15mins   30mins   hourly
Postcode   Tel No.   self return

Age   D.O.B.   Next of Kin (if applicable)
Name
Occupation   Religion   Address

G.P.   Tel No.

Date of Arrival   Relatives Informed   Yes   No

Time of Arrival   Present Yes No

Nursing Assessment (Abdominal/G.I. Related Conditions)

History. Date of Onset   Time of Onset   Trauma Related Yes No
(Include all relevant past medical/social history) if RTA driver/passenger/
pedestrian

Fig. 7/5   A & E card; first section

Conscious State: Full   Disorientated/confused   Drowsy

Human Behaviour State: Relaxed   Anxious   Aggressive
                        Hysterical   Disruptive

Pain: Nil   Mild   Severe   Unbearable

Description

Position

Radiating   Yes/No   Pain in back   Yes/No
            Where

Non Verbal Signs   Is abdomen distended   Yes/No

Related to food   Yes/No   Relived by medication   Yes/No
What   What

Relieved by position   Yes/No
What

Skin Colour/Temp.: Pale   Cyanosed   Flushed   Normal
                    Cold   Hot   Wet   Dry

Resp. Rate   Rhythm   Pulse Rate   Rhythm   B.P.
                    Temp.

Wound   Yes/No   Site   Dehydration   Yes/No

Nausea   Yes/No   Vomiting   Yes/No   Consistence   Amount

Urine: Burning/Frenquency/Retention
        Difficulty/Incontinence/Normal

Bladder: Distended   Yes/No   Urine Test

Bowels: Constipated   Diarrhoea   Normal

Faeces: Colour   Consistence

Weight Loss   Yes/No   L.M.P.

Fluid/Blood Loss   P.R.   Yes/No   P.V.   Yes/No

Fig. 7/6   A & E card; second section

Where additional problems are identified the add-on cards allow
for more detailed assessment of the situation, e.g. chief complaint:
limb injury. If a wound was also present on the limb then the wound

add-on card would be used in addition to the chief complaint record (Fig. 7/7).

Where many add-on cards would be required, e.g. multiply injured patients, a specific card should be created. Adapted versions of the chief complaint cards allow for unnecessary documentation to be removed when the nurse is dealing with a relatively minor problem.

Wound Add-on Card

Airway: Clear   Obstructed

Estimated Blood Loss   Type of Bleeding

Cause of Wound (if bullet high or low velocity)

Area of Damage

Is Wound: Clean   Dirty   Clean cut   Jagged
                 Bite (human/animal)

Tissue Loss   Yes No   Amount

Depth of Wound   Any Swelling   Yes No

Any F.B.   Yes No   Pulse Distal to Injury   Yes No

Any obvious underlying damage to bone/tendon/vessels/organs
    Yes No

Nursing Intervention

Temporary dressing applied   Type

If upper limbs. Rings removed   Yes No N/A

Tetanus immunisation given   Yes No   Start of course   Booster

---

Fig. 7/7   Wound add-on card

Section three identifies the intervention stage of care (Fig. 7/8). Intervention, like the assessment stage of care, must be recorded. Although patients with the same problems will have specific intervention, it was found more difficult to pre-record intervention in

---

Nursing Intervention

Patient made comfortable on bed/trolley   Yes No   Area of Dept

Position on bed/trolley

Nil by Mouth   Yes No   Vomit bowls and tissues given   Yes No
Mouth washes provided   Yes No

<u>Further Intervention</u>   <u>Signature</u>

Fig. 7/8   A & E card; third section

the same way as for assessment. Where this was possible, pre-
printing of the intervention stage is made available on the record
card.

A large area is also available for specific intervention to be
recorded, individual to that patient. Recording of intervention carried out, following the medical staff's prescription, is identified by
the nurse signing and putting the time of intervention against the

prescribed care, e.g. the doctor prescribes a drug, the nurse signs the card and puts the time the drug was given.

Section four is a blank A4 section which allows medical documentation to take place and the final section provides for evaluation (Fig. 7/9). The evaluation section is pre-printed on the back of the card. It allows the nurse to identify whether planned care has been achieved and if the patient is being discharged, what instructions and discharge advice cards have been given. It also allows for an indication of what community services have been arranged. If the patient is being admitted, an area on the evaluation record records property taken with the patient to the ward.

Evaluation

How is patient's condition now?   Have the goals been achieved?

ADMISSION		DISCHARGE
Ward	Time to Ward	Self Care instructions given
		Yes No
Clothes	In property bag	
	Given to relative/friend	Specifiy
Dentures	None	
	In PTS mouth	
	In denture pot	Follow up/OPD appt given
	Given to relatives/friend	Yes No
Spectacles	None	
	PT wearing	
	In property bag	
	Given to relatives/friend	
Valuables	None	
	Handed in for safe keeping	
	With PT	
	Given to relatives/friend	
Other aids		

Nurse completing evaluation_ _

Fig. 7/9   A & E card; final section

PLANNING CARE

Accident and Emergency trained nurses should know, based on their knowledge and the assessment conducted, the care patients require. This knowledge and the skill of patient assessment, should be part of a total development package in any A & E unit. Policy and procedure manuals, general guidelines and the availability of nursing and medical books should provide the nurse with the ability to plan patient care.

In addition patient assessment and care planning should, in A & E, only be undertaken by senior staff with more junior staff, learning through experience. Following this philosophy and the reality of care being provided soon after the assessment stage, it is unnecessary for the record form to provide large areas for planned care, but it does require detailed documentation of the nursing intervention. Often the intervention reflects the plan that would have been made in the nurse's head. Planned re-assessment must be identified and recorded and obviously any planned care for a period of time, must also be documented.

PROBLEMS

Both potential and actual problems will have been identified. Actual problems will be reflected in the particular card the triage nurse has chosen. Further problems will be reflected in the use of add-on cards or the record of assessment. Potential problems will be reflected more in the documentation of the intervention rather than requiring a separate area on the record card e.g. the recording of the use of cot sides in the intervention stage reflects that the nurse identified a potential problem of the patient falling out of the bed/trolley.

PRIORITY RATING AND DEPENDENCY SCALE

This must be recorded and a space is available on the front of the form.

GOALS

Specific goals will reflect in the documentation at the intervention stage, e.g. a wound that is bleeding profusely creates a specific goal of preventing further blood loss. The planned care is to provide a temporary pressure dressing. The intervention is to apply that dressing. It is reasonable, therefore, to assume that if the record of assessment indicates a wound bleeding profusely and the record of intervention shows a pressure dressing was applied, then the nurse must have identified a specific goal, planned the care and thus intervened.

Further examples of planning being reflected in the assessment and intervention records

Assessment – Patient is suffering from a wrist injury ? fracture. The assessment of the limb indicates swelling, deformity and pain – *this is recorded.*

In the nurse's head *unrecorded* the potential problem of obstructed blood flow to the hand is considered. Radial pulse is felt and is present – *this is recorded.* The recording of the pulse being present shows that the nurse considered the potential problem of obstructed blood flow, planned to assess the pulse and recorded her findings.

While continuing the care, the nurse identifies a goal to reduce the swelling. She plans to use ice packs and elevation – this goal and planning is *unrecorded* but in the intervention stage of care, the use of ice-pack and elevated sling, *which has been recorded*, clearly identifies that the planning stage took place.

Reassessment of the pulse is required every half hour; this plan is recorded because it needs to be seen by other staff so they can continue the care.

The patient lives alone and may require home help. This pre-planning is reflected in the intervention record, by indicating that social workers have been contacted. If further notification of social workers is required at a later stage of care, this would be recorded as further intervention required.

By using an integrated medical/nursing record, documentation of patient care within the A & E department is kept to a minimum, but ensures all three essential reasons for documenting care are achieved. The record card acts as a legal document and an educational tool which provides guidance and instruction and reflects the care given.

Summary

The one area of nursing that concerns a large number of Accident and Emergency nurses is the need to document the care provided. Nurses still resist the introduction of nursing records into the department, and generally record as little as possible. Various reasons can be suggested for this reluctance. It is probably due chiefly to non-accident and emergency nurses attempting to implement ward systems into the department rather than accident nurses developing documents that would suit themselves, provide the necessary information, but still be useable during the busy as well as the quiet periods.

The documentation recommended provides a clear system of recording all aspects of the process of Accident and Emergency care but allows the nurse to achieve a concise record with the minimum of writing.

PART THREE

The Process in Action

8 *Case histories*

In the first two parts of this book the process of care in A & E has been discussed. It is now possible to use the process to follow through the complete care of patients with individual problems that present every day in the A & E department. A comparison will be made, where appropriate, between a patient following care in a logical, structured manner, and one that with similar problems who is not.

Case one

Miss Green is an elderly lady of 86 years. Throughout her life she had been independent and was still very active in both mind and body. Miss Green fell and fractured her left wrist. She also bruised her left shin and knee, quite extensively. The injury to her leg created great difficulty with walking, especially when bending the leg.

CARE WITHOUT A STRUCTURED APPROACH

Miss Green arrived in the A & E department at 2 p.m. on a Friday afternoon. She was brought into the department by a neighbour and was helped out of the car by the porter and placed in a wheelchair. At reception Miss Green, although in some degree of pain, typically did not make an issue of her injury and spoke quite cheerfully to the receptionist. She dismissed the neighbour, saying she would call him when she was ready to return home. Once registered, Miss Green was pushed into the waiting room and the A & E card put through to the clinical area. At 3 p.m. Miss Green was seen by the A & E S.H.O. and diagnosed as possibly having a fracture of her left wrist and bruising to the left knee and shin. She was sent to

X-ray. At 3.30 p.m. Miss Green arrived back in the department and at 4 p.m. was seen again. Undisplaced fracture of the lower end of radius was diagnosed and a plaster of Paris prescribed, as was Tubigrip to her left knee and shin and analgesia. She was discharged, to be followed up in the fracture clinic.

Miss Green was taken to the plaster room and a plaster of Paris applied. She was then returned to the dressing area for the Tubigrip. At 4.15 p.m. the neighbour was asked to return and on arrival at 5.15 p.m. attempted to get Miss Green in his car. The leg was very painful and Miss Green had difficulty in bending the knee. At this stage problems began to emerge:

1 Miss Green lived on the second floor in a set of flats without a lift.
2 She was left handed with a very weak right hand.
3 She had no relatives.
4 The social work department closed at 4.30 p.m.

An ambulance was booked to take Miss Green home. The neighbour said he would see Miss Green into her flat. The nurse said social services would be contacted on Monday morning about home help and meals on wheels. Miss Green departed.

Discussion

Without a structured approach to the care a number of potential problems, both social and physical, had been missed on arrival. No logical approach to the assessment had been undertaken, other than a medical assessment based on the presenting problem. Intervention had been based purely on the medical presentation, and diagnosis and evaluation of the care was impossible to achieve.

Arrival – No triage system was in operation. No nursing assessment was performed. Distal circulation to the limb could have been impaired. No thought was given to discharge.

Assessment and intervention – Purely based on the injury and medical diagnosis.

Discharge – Only at this stage were problems about the social situation identified.

CARE USING THE PROCESS OF CARE

Arrival – Having arrived in the department, Miss Green would have been seen by the triage nurse, either before or immediately after registration. The triage nurse would have welcomed Miss Green and with the use of the model of nursing commenced the first-stage assessment.

Communication

This would give rise to the beginning of the partnership between the triage nurse and Miss Green. During the initial discussion, the triage nurse would have seen clearly that no problem existed with the airway, breathing or circulatory component. However, she would have assessed the radial pulse distal to the arm injury and the colour and movement of the fingers. The leg would have likewise been assessed and the bruising identified. During the communication, it would have been established that Miss Green was left-handed and her personal care and environmental safety would have been identified. The lack of lift facilities at her home would also have been noted. It would have also been identified that problems with cooking, washing and dressing were going to be present. The lack of mobility in the knee would have been assessed. The last meal and drink would have been recorded at this stage.

Problems – actual

1 Left wrist injury ? Fracture.
2 Left leg and knee injury.
3 Lives in second floor flat, no lift.
4 Left-handed, weak right hand.

Potential problems

1 Unable to get up stairs to flat.
2 Unable to wash and dress adequately.
3 Unable to cook, without risk of dropping pans, etc.

Further communication would have identified that Miss Green had no relatives and was going to find life very difficult, when discharged.

Intervention – pre-medical care
The injured arm would have been placed in a sling. A leg elevator is used to support the injured leg. Ice-packs would have been applied to the knee to reduce swelling, thus attempting to retain movement. Miss Green would have been advised to remain nil by mouth.

Non-medical nursing care
With Miss Green's permission, the social work department and community liaison nurses would have been contracted and asked to visit during Miss Green's A & E stay. Although the social work department may not have been able to organize any assistance over the weekend, services could have been up and ready on Monday morning. The community liaison nurses would be able to organize an evening service to commence that day. Medical intervention would not have changed and treatment would not have altered. Timing would have been the same. Once medical, nursing and social intervention were complete, an ambulance would have been organized for Miss Green's discharge, having first discussed with the neighbour support over the weekend.

Evaluation

It is possible to evaluate the care given because a logical process of care had been implemented. The left wrist was fractured and placed in plaster of Paris. The left leg and knee was bruised. Swelling had been minimized due to the use of ice-packs and movement, although slightly difficult, was not impossible. The social worker had organized meals on wheels and home help to commence on Monday morning. The community liaison nurse had organized a service from that evening to help Miss Green undress, wash and get to bed. The neighbours had agreed to help Miss Green over the weekend with meals, etc. The ambulance transport arrived and discharge was achieved.

Case two

CARE WITHOUT A STRUCTURED APPROACH

Mr Thompson was a 45-year-old man. On Sunday morning he registered at the desk and sat in the waiting room. On the accident and emergency card the receptionist had written sore throat. General comments regarding the use of A & E were made by the staff on duty and no further consideration was given to Mr Thompson until called through to see the doctor. During the medical examination Mr Thompson gave a history of pain in the throat coming on suddenly at 5 a.m. that morning. He appeared slightly pale and was very anxious. Various investigations were recommended and following these a diagnosis of myocardial infarction was made. Mr Thompson was admitted.

Discussion

Mr Thompson had sat in a waiting-room having suffered a serious cardiac problem. Had there been a structured process of care within A & E this would not have occurred. During the triage stage of the patient's care, the nurse would have established through communication, the difference between what Mr Thompson was calling a sore throat and what was actually pain in the throat. Further communication would have established that the pain suddenly came at 5 a.m. and woke him. The slight pallor of the skin would also have been noted and also during the assessment of the airway, breathing and circulation component, the pulse and blood pressure recording may well have assisted in the overall picture.

Nursing intervention could have been based on a much more structured approach with the patient being taken to a cubicle and further in-depth assessment and care being performed. The potential cardiac problem would have been identified. Priority rating and patient dependency would have been determined and appropriate medical and nursing intervention carried out.

The two cases presented show clearly how the lack of a process of care in A & E can lead to inadequate patient assessment, due to:

1 No triage system.
2 No structure (model) to follow.

The following case histories are presented using the process.

Case three

SPINAL INJURY

Mr Smith was unloading his lorry when he fell back and landed on a bar. The metal bar struck him across the lower section of the posterior wall of the chest. Mr Smith lay, unable to get up from his fallen position.

Arrival in A & E

The triage nurse was given a full history of events from the ambulance personnel. When meeting Mr Smith, the triage nurse performed a first-stage assessment.

Communication

Mr Smith was conscious and complaining of pain in his back across the lower section of the chest. Mr Smith was anxious and concerned that his wife was unaware of his accident. Mr Smith has no previous medical history. Touch sensation to the lower limbs was absent.

Airway, breathing, circulation

Airway and breathing was not affected by the injury. Pulse was 75 beats per minute regular and blood pressure was 150/70 mm Hg. Skin colour was normal.

Mobility

The patient arrived on a stretcher. The ambulance crew had placed a cervical collar on Mr Smith and supported his legs together with triangular slings. He was lying on a spinal board.

Eating, drinking, elimination

Mr Smith did not complain of any gastro-intestinal or genito-urinary problems.

Personal care

The patient had old, work clothes on and the skin of the face and hands was dirty.

Environmental safety and health promotion

The injury was due to a work-related accident.

SPECIFIC IN-DEPTH ASSESSMENT

This took place in the major treatment cubicle and was performed by the primary nurse. Mr Smith had been placed on an all-purpose care trolley.

Communication

A full history was obtained as to the exact mode of injury. Mr Smith explained clearly that while pulling at a rope he fell and struck his back across a metal bar. He did not strike his head. Mr Smith complained of pain at the site of injury but his lower body felt heavy. No alcohol or drugs had been taken.

Human behaviour

Mr Smith was anxious about his injury and also about his wife not being aware of his accident. He co-operated well and a partnership was developing between him and the primary nurse.

Physiological senses
The loss of sensation was quite marked in the lower limbs. Slight 'pins and needles' could be described from the right foot.

Mobility

Mr Smith was able to move his arms. He was unable to move his legs. No attempt was made to turn or allow Mr Smith to move further.

PROBLEMS – ACTUAL (A), POTENTIAL (P)

1 Pain in the lower thoracic spine (A).
2 Inability to move legs (A).
3 Inability to feel touch/sensation in legs (A).
4 Anxiety (A).
5 Spinal damage (P).
6 Retention of urine (P).
7 Pressure sores (P).
8 Other organ damage, e.g. spleen (P).

SPECIFIC GOALS

1 Prevent any movement of spine.
2 Support the legs and neck.
3 Reduce the anxiety.
4 Reduce the risk of pressure sore development.
5 Allow urine to be eliminated.

Priority rating – URGENT (2). Patient dependency – HIGH DEPENDENCY (2).

INTERVENTION

Communication

Mr Smith was told that he may have damaged his back and until medical examination and X-ray had been taken, all movement was to be restricted. Mr Smith's wife was contacted and he was told she was on her way to the department.

Mobility

Because of the potential spinal damage, Mr Smith's clothes were cut and removed leaving them *in situ* where it was impossible, without rolling him, to remove them from the trolley. The cervical collar was left *in situ* ensuring areas where pressure to the skin was present were padded. The legs were support with sandbags.

Airway, breathing, circulation

Regular vital signs were recorded.

Eating, drinking, elimination

A catheterization trolley was prepared.

MEDICAL INTERVENTION

A full medical assessment, including X-rays, was undertaken. The catheter was passed and urine obtained.

Mobility/personal care

During the medical assessment, Mr Smith was log rolled. This procedure was performed using four nurses. As Mr Smith was rolled his cut clothing was removed and sheepskin placed under his back and buttocks in the effort to prevent pressure sore development. Sheepskin bootees were also put on his heels.

EVALUATION

Mr Smith had a spinal injury and required admission. Accident and emergency care had prevented any further damage.

Movement of the spine had been reduced with the continued use

of the care trolley, cervical collar and support of legs. No movement of the patient had occurred without a full team of medical
and nursing personnel being present and then the log roll was
used.

Mr Smith's anxiety had been reduced by:

1 Explaining each stage of care and developing a partnership
between him and the primary nurse.
2 The arrival of Mrs Smith.

Pressure sore development had been reduced by the use of
sheepskins on the trolley and the removal of Mr Smith's clothing.

Urine was able to be eliminated due to the catheter insertion.
No potential nursing problems had become actual problems and
Mr Smith left the department to continue his care on the ward.

Case four

John arrived in the accident and emergency department in a very
disruptive state. He was shouting, swearing and with great
strength attempting to get off the ambulance stretcher. Two
ambulance crews were in attendance and when seen by the triage
nurse, John was immediately sent to a clinical room which was
isolated from the main treatment area. Several nurses and porters
assisted in the room, while the primary nurse began a nursing
assessment.

COMMUNICATION

The ambulance crew had been called to a meeting spot, used by
the local youths. No one in the area could give any information.
The ambulance crew suspected either drugs, glue or possibly a
hypoglycaemic attack, but had been unable to find any medic alert.
John was exhibiting very violent, but confused behaviour. He did
not appear to know what was happening.

AIRWAY, BREATHING, CIRCULATION

John's skin was slightly pale and moist. All systems appeared normal. It was impossible to obtain an accurate pulse rate or blood pressure.

MOBILITY

Very active, thrashing all limbs – required restraint.

EATING, DRINKING, ELIMINATION

With effort a blood (fingerprick) specimen was achieved and a blood glucose level obtained. It was very low (1 mmol/l).

PERSONAL CARE

Looked well-dressed, skin was clean.

ENVIRONMENTAL SAFETY AND HEALTH PROMOTION

With the physical and mental state that John was displaying, a high risk existed for his safety. He was restrained by nursing and portering staff in a room that was away from the main treatment area.

PROBLEM

1 Very agitated and disruptive (A).
2 Risk of personal harm (A).
3 Hypoglycaemia (A).
4 Unconsciousness (P).
5 Injury from restraint (P).

GOALS

1 Return blood sugar to normal.

2 Prevent injury to patient and staff.

3 Achieve the return of John's self-care and independence.

Priority rating – IMMEDIATE (1). Dependency – TOTAL (1).

INTERVENTION

Communication

Although John did not appear to understand what was happening, it was essential to keep talking to him and requesting his co-operation.

Mobility

Restraint was provided to ensure he did not injure himself. Restraint was by physical support rather than any straps. Staff allowed some controlled movements. This prevented injury to John from muscle contraction, without movement.

Eating, drinking, elimination

I.V. glucose was given by the A & E S.H.O. After a short period the glucose was active and the blood sugar level increased.

EVALUATION

John became quiet. He lay still for some time and then spoke rationally. He asked where he was and what had happened. He admitted suffering from diabetes (insulin dependent) but did not carry any identification. He had not eaten any lunch.

The blood sugar and therefore consciousness and human behavioural state had returned to normal. No physical harm had occurred to either John or the staff.

John had returned to self-care. However, he received a long explanation from the primary nurse regarding the correct care of his diabetes. This was followed up with a request from the nurse to the

diabetic liaison officer to visit John, prior to discharge. This result-
ed in John going home, knowing that follow-up visits from the
diabetic liaison officer would occur.

Case five

Mrs Stephens was 35. She had suffered from inoperable stomach
cancer for some time. Cytotoxic therapy had been unsuccessful and
terminal care had been provided at home. Today Mr Stephens
became frightened as his wife was having difficulty swallowing and
was becoming unconscious. Despite wishing for death to occur in
the family home, Mr Stephens rang for an ambulance, as today he
was on his own and did not feel able to cope. Mrs Stephens started
vomiting and was incontinent of both urine and faeces.

On arrival in accident and emergency, Mrs Stephens was
allocated a bed rather than a trolley. The triage nurse recognized at
once that comfort for both Mr and Mrs Stephens was the top
priority. The primary nurse assigned to Mrs Stephens, made a full
first- and second-stage assessment.

COMMUNICATION

Communication with both Mr and Mrs Stephens was essential and
it was important that Mr Stephens was not excluded from any care.
Mr Stephens felt he had lost the final wish for his wife to die at
home. It was essential the nurse helped him see the logic in calling
for help.

AIRWAY, BREATHING, CIRCULATION

Airway care was maintained by positioning Mrs Stephens on her
side. Regular mouth toilet was provided. Breathing was very weak
and shallow. Circulation was poor.

MOBILITY

Mrs Stephens, although still conscious but very drowsy, was not able to move, other than to hold her husband's hand. This was encouraged by the nurse.

EATING, DRINKING, ELIMINATION

Constant attention was provided to keep the bed clean and the skin dry. Air fresheners were placed discreetly in the room to remove the faecal odour.

PERSONAL CARE

Personal care was of paramount importance. Although Mrs Stephens had not long to spend before death, personal care was given. Mr Stephens wished to help with the care and he was encouraged to do so. Mrs Stephens died within 1 hour of arriving in the Accident and Emergency department. Mr Stephens was devastated, despite the preparation of some weeks. The primary nurse continued care of Mr Stephens, while other nurses attended to Mrs Stephens.

COMMUNICATION

This component of life becomes very important for relatives at such a time as sudden death. Mr Stephens began talking of the past. The happy times the two had had together. The primary nurse listened and said nothing. Mr Stephens cried. The primary nurse held his hand. Mr Stephens talked about the death. The primary nurse listened and supported verbally, when necessary. Mr Stephens asked 'What happens now?' The primary nurse explained.

DISCUSSION

Despite Mrs Stephens dying in the accident and emergency department rather than at home, Mr Stephens was not alone. He had the support, the partnership of one other person. He was able to share in the last moments of his wife's life and was able to see she was comfortable and well cared for. The process of care, because it provides a structured approach, an individual approach, allowed for the death, although sad, to be dignified.

The triage nurse, having performed a first-stage assessment, identified the need for terminal nursing care, therefore a bed not a trolley was used. A primary nurse took Mr and Mrs Stephens together and treated them as one. The second-stage assessment identified specific problems that required nursing intervention and it was clear that when death occurred, the nursing intervention had to continue for Mr Stephens. All physical and psychological care was provided for both Mr and Mr Stephens and the death was therefore achieved in a dignified manner and in such a way that Mr Stephens could now continue his grieving process.

9 The process in education

All accident and emergency departments need to educate trained staff who are new to the department. Most departments also have a commitment to learner training. The process of care allows for education of both trained and student nurses in a logical manner. The structured approach, through the assessment, problem identification, goal setting, intervention and evaluation stages of the process provides new nurses with a framework to follow. The model allows the nurse to take each component of life and identify its link with the stages of the process.

Starting at the beginning

The most sensible way of educating staff new to the A & E department is to use an orientation programme. The nurse must be made aware of the A & E philosophy. Discussion should take place regarding what is meant by health and quality of life, the independence and dignity that should be shown to all patients and how freedom of choice must be balanced with the need for care.

Health, as defined by the World Health Organization, is a state of complete physical, mental and social well-being and not merely the absence of disease. No allowance is made within this definition for variation. It would seem to suggest a situation in which one has either health or ill-health and begs the question as to how many people could be categorized as healthy if the criteria is strictly interpreted.

The well person usually has some small degree of physical or mental illness and a person who is approaching death may still have some health potential. To some extent this health–illness continuum has been addressed by nurses in allocating dependency levels. Nurses have a responsibility to the clients to facilitate the optimum state of health through example and active participation in health education.

Quality of life – The suggestion is that quality relates to individuals obtaining a sense of satisfaction with the level of physical, emotional and social comfort which they experience. The standard of quality is determined through the individual's own perception. The nurse's responsibility therefore relates to attempting to meet the individuals' perceived needs for quality in their life. This is sometimes difficult due to the patient's pre-conceived ideas and expectations not always being met.

New nursing staff must be prepared for this problem.

The model

The A & E model of nursing lends itself to the education of all nursing staff. Each component of life is a major educational tool in itself.

COMMUNICATION

Communication skills must be developed during the orientation period. Various aspects of communication must be considered including in-depth reference to children, elderly, mentally disturbed, suddenly bereaved relatives and to specific physiological and human behavioural problems.

The new nurse through experiential methods, guidance from senior staff (mentor) and group discussion with their peers, will:

1 Participate in encouraging effective communication in A & E by:
   (a) Relaying information between members of the team.
   (b) Ensuring all printed information is made available on notice boards, communication books, etc.
2 Develop communication skills, empathy and reassurance skills, as relevant to families of patients who are being treated in the A & E setting.
3 Demonstrate increased confidence when interviewing individuals/families of all ages and obtaining the history of injury/ill health.

4 Examine their own attitudes/non-verbal communication to both staff and patients and their ability to establish a good rapport with both.

5 Demonstrate increased confidence in communicating with patients of varying behavioural levels, including those with altered body image.

6 Discuss society's and health workers' views of the elderly.

7 Develop an insight into social and psychological effects of orthopaedic, medical and surgical conditions, including trauma, both to the patient and relatives.

8 Discuss sociological and demographic factors affecting attendance in the A & E department.

9 Demonstrate an understanding and use of the Coma Scale.

10 Demonstrate the correct method of examining patients with eye conditions.

11 Discuss the various ways pain is demonstrated by the patient.

12 Discuss legal and ethical implications of sudden death.

13 Develop sensitive understanding of the practical and emotional issues, surrounding dying and bereavement.

14 Discuss the effect of death of a child on the family and other siblings.

AIRWAY, BREATHING, CIRCULATION

Knowledge of the anatomy and the physiology of the respiratory and circulatory system will have been provided during nurse training. New nurses should be required to demonstrate skills necessary to assess and observe the individual, when establishing vital signs and base line observations and to meet the individual's airway, breathing and circulatory needs.

The new nurse should through guidance, from senior staff, lectures, videos and experience:

1 Extend her knowledge of shock.

2 Develop greater ability to apply knowledge of shock to nursing management.

3 Analyse the use of trauma and injury severity scores and their contribution to effective management of patients.

4 Give effective total management of patients with airway, breathing or circulatory collapse:
   (a) Airway obstruction.
   (b) Respiratory arrest.
   (c) Cardiac arrest.
5 Become proficient in the recording of ECG's and interpretations of arrhythmias.
6 Develop the skill of I.V. cannulation and fluid replacement.
7 Discuss the effects of trauma on homeostasis.

MOBILITY

The degree of dependence a patient has on a nurse tends to relate to the level of mobility which a patient can obtain. Many patients in accident and emergency require limbs to be held immobile and the nurse must be aware of the various splints available. The new nurse should, through guidance from senior staff, lectures, videos and experience:

1 Be able to demonstrate the correct use of various splints available.
2 Be able to demonstrate the correct use of appropriate lifting techniques and the equipment used.
3 Be able to discuss the effect of immobility in relation to pressure sore risk.
4 Be able to demonstrate assessment techniques required to identify a patient's mobility status.
5 Be able to discuss the effect immobility has in relation to age.
6 Be able to demonstrate the correct care of patients with potential spinal injury.

EATING, DRINKING, ELIMINATION

The knowledge of changes in a patient's fluid and electrolyte balance and gastrointestinal activity following sudden illness or trauma, allows the nurse to meet the individuals nutritional needs and fluid and electrolyte replacement. Through guidance from senior staff, group discussion, lectures, videos and experience the A & E nurse should be able to:

1 Discuss the need for many patients in A & E to be kept nil by mouth.
2 Demonstrate the correct methods of removing poisonous substances from the patient's stomach.
3 Demonstrate the correct method of obtaining a blood sugar result at departmental level.
4 Demonstrate the technique of urinary catheterisation.

ENVIRONMENTAL SAFETY AND HEALTH PROMOTION

Safety of both patients and staff is important. The accident and emergency environment must reflect the nurse's attitude to safety and health promotion. The nurse must, through visits to health promotional departments, by studying attendances in accident and emergency and by reading legal documentation (e.g. Health & Safety at Work Act) be able to:

1 Extend awareness of the role which they as individuals can perform.
2 Be aware of and value the facilities/agencies and materials available to enable them to promote health.
3 Review current health promotional activities and consider ways in which they can be made more effective.
4 Analyse their own attitude to Health Promotion and endeavour to develop a healthier lifestyle.
5 Develop further skills in promoting health.
6 Appreciate ways in which the knowledge/attitude to health influences accident and emergency attendance.
7 Extend their understanding of the role of occupational health nurses.
8 Consider the topic of stress and its affect on health in the working environment.
9 Extend their awareness of specific environmental influences on health in the local catchment area.
10 Appreciate the affect of radiation and X-rays.
11 Correctly dispose of contaminated infected material.
12 Discuss responsibility for the maintenance of safety and prevention of injury and accident.
13 Outline and adhere to health and safety policies relating to work in the unit.

14 Debate issues arising from Health & Safety at Work Act.
15 Become proficient in the action to be taken in the event of fire, bomb alert, or a major incident call being activated.

PERSONAL CARE

Like mobility, the amount of personal care the patient requires will depend largely on the dependency the patient has on the nurse:

1 The nurse should be aware of facilities available for personal care in the A & E department and in the community.
2 The correct care of patients valuables and clothing.
3 The correct disposal of linen.

Triage including patient dependency for nursing intervention

New nurses must be provided with the opportunity under expert guidance to extend their understanding of triage and develop the ability to apply the priority rating with greater accuracy. The development of algorithms by the new nurse, with senior guidance, allows for discussion. A base line algorithm can be reviewed at intervals during the orientation programme and changes made. Role play in groups can also help develop the nurse's ability to triage more effectively.

DEPENDENCY

The use of the dependency rating scale is a major help when developing the nurse's judgemental skills (see Table 3/2). The nurse is able to take each component of life and when assessing the patient, can make a comparison between a number of variables. By adding the number from each component of life, a dependency score can be achieved. As the nurse's knowledge and judgemental skills develop, the use of the scale will become automatic.

10 *Self-evaluation*

This chapter allows you to evaluate your theoretical skills of A & E nursing. A number of patients will be introduced to you. You will be asked questions throughout the chapter regarding these patients and you can check your answers with those provided.

Patient 1

A 35-year-old male patient is admitted to the accident and emergency department complaining of abdominal pain. What do you want to know during your assessment?

Patient 2

An 18-year-old male patient arrives in the accident and emergency department complaining of a wrist injury. What do you want to know during your assessment?

Patient 3

A 45-year-old lady arrives unconscious. What immediate action would you take? What dependency rating would she deserve?

Patient 4

An 85-year-old lady has been brought into accident and emergency by her son. He says she cannot cope at home any longer. Where do you begin?

Patient 5

A 35-year-old male, manual worker, arrives in the department complaining of pain with a foreign body in his right eye. Describe your assessment.

Patient 1

- The patient's name is John.
- He lives locally with his parents.
- He is unemployed.
- He is fully conscious and alert, he is anxious and in pain.
- The pain came on 2 hours ago. It is central and described as stabbing in nature. It radiates to the right iliac fossa. There is no pain in the back and the abdomen is not distended.
- Diet, medication and position do not affect the pain.
- Skin colour is normal.
- Respiration rate is 16. Pulse is 80 and regular. Blood pressure is 130/75 mm Hg. Temperature is 38°C.
- There is no abdominal wound. John is not dehydrated.
- Nausea is present and vomiting occurred prior to arrival.
- Bladder and bowels are normal. No weight or fluid loss has occurred.

Patient 2

- The patient's name is Mark.
- He lives on his own in a flat.
- He works as a labourer on the local building site.
- He is fully conscious and alert. He is reasonably relaxed.
- He has quite severe pain in his wrist. There is no loss of sensation/motor deficit.
- Skin colour of the hand and wrist is normal.
- The radical pulse is present. Swelling is present.
- Slight deformity is seen. Mark cannot move his wrist without severe pain.

- He last ate 2 hours ago, but had a cup of tea after the injury, to calm his nerves.

Patient 3

- Care of the airway would be paramount.
- The lady would be placed on her side.
- Suction if necessary, would be used to remove any excess saliva.
- The jaw would be positioned to establish an open airway.
- A full examination of the lady, from head to toe, would be undertaken.
- Vital signs would be recorded. A blood sugar test would be performed.
- ECG recording would be undertaken.
- The lady would be undressed. Any identification, medic alert, etc. would be noted. Dependency rating would be total (1).

Patient 4

- The patients name is Mrs Annie Smith.
- She lives alone in a four-bedroomed house.
- The toilet and bathroom are upstairs.
- Mrs Smith is conscious but confused.
- There does not appear to be a chief complaint, but the son, who lives 200 miles away, insists she can no longer cope at home.
- From general observation, Mrs Smith appears to be hard of hearing and her sight is diminished.
- She does not appear to be in pain.
- Her airway, breathing and circulation appear stable.
- Mrs Smith is able to walk, but is very unstable on her feet.
- Eating, drinking, elimination components appear unaffected, although the skin does suggest slight dehydration.
- The furred tongue also suggests lack of fluid intake.
- Mrs Smith is unwashed and clothes are soiled. A slight body odour exists. The son states that his mother can no longer get

upstairs to the toilet. She uses a bucket in the lounge and empties this down the drain outside. She attempts to wash in the kitchen, but recently has appeared to have stopped this activity.

Patient 5

- The patient's name is Steven.
- He is married and drives a car.
- He works on a building site and was breaking up some cement slabs with a sledge hammer.
- Steven is very anxious and complaining of severe pain in the right eye.
- A high-velocity foreign body is probably present.
- Eye examination reveals:
  Left eye:
    Visual acuity 6/6.
    Lids normal.
    Conjunctiva normal.
    Cornea normal.
    Anterior chamber present.
    Pupil regular, central and reactive.
    Globe normal.
  Right Eye:
    Visual Acuity 6/60.
    Lids red from rubbing.
    Conjunctiva injected.
    Cornea misty.
    Anterior chamber shallow? Flat.
    Pupil dilated and fixed.
    Globe normal.

Patients 2 and 4

1 What problems do you identify (actual and potential)?

2 What goals do you set?
3 What intervention prior to medical care do you perform?

Patient 3

What probable causes can you list which may be the reason for the patient's unconscious state?

Patient 5

1 What is the probable injury to Steven's eye?
2 What care would you give prior to medical intervention?

Mark (Patient 2).

PROBLEMS

Actual

1 Wrist injury ? Fracture
2 Pain severe

Potential

1 May require anaesthetic for manipulation.
2 May have problem with circulation to the hand.
3 Will not be able to work for some weeks.
4 May need assistance with housework/cooking.

GOALS

1 Support of limb.
2 Reduction in pain.
3 Reduction of swelling.

4 Keeping the stomach empty (nil by mouth)
5 Providing advice on assistance if required.

INTERVENTION

1 Arm sling applied ⎫
                   ⎬ helps reduce pain
2 Ice-packs to wrist ⎭
3 Priority rating URGENT.
4 Advised to remain Nil by Mouth.
5 Radial pulse monitored regularly.
6 Social worker contacted re. advice on sickness pay and assistance.

Mrs Smith (Patient 4)

PROBLEMS

Actual

1 Lives alone. Toilet and bathroom upstairs.
2 Confused. Hard of hearing.
3 Poor sight.
4 Unstable on feet.
5 Slight dehydration.
6 Personal care poor.

Potential

1 Further dehydration/malnutrition.
2 Environmentally unsafe:
   (a) Falls.
   (b) Infection.
   (c) Lack of health care.
   (d) Further lack of personal care.
   (e) Confused state could cause fires.
3 Hypothermia.
4 Skin breakdown to pressure sores.

Goals

1 Identify how independent Mrs Smith can become.
2 Ensure Mrs Smith is environmentally safe in the A & E department.
3 Improve hydration.
4 Improve personal care.
5 Involve social services/community services.
6 Dependency rating – high.

INTERVENTION

Before providing personal care, ask the S.H.O. to have a brief look at Mrs Smith. This allows the S.H.O. to be aware of the presenting condition should admission/discharge be in dispute at a later time.

Provide personal care, bedbath, clean gown, mouth, hair and nail care.

Unless there is any contra-indication, provide fluids and light diet. Ensure son or nurse observes Mrs Smith at all times. Cot sides on the bed may be necessary, but can cause further confusion in the elderly. Speak loudly and clearly. Keep near to Mrs Smith so she can see you. Alert social services department. Discuss further care with son.

Patient No. 3

1 Head injury.
2 Overdose.
3 Neurological disorder, e.g. cerebral bleed, subarachnoid haemorrhage.
4 Hypoglycaemic coma.
5 Post-epileptic fit.
6 Stoke-Adams attack.
7 Asphyxia.
8 Other metabolic disorders.

Steven, Patient 5

1 Probable injury.
2 High-velocity foreign body (piece of cement slab).
3 Perforated cornea and now intraocular foreign body exists.
4 Lens may have sustained a traumatic cataract.

PRE-MEDICAL CARE

1 Steven would be taken to the examination room and laid flat.
2 A temporary eye pad would be applied. Steven would be advised not to bend forward.
3 Priority rating would be immediate.

Patient 6

Julie is 6 years old. She lives with her mother and her stepfather. Julie arrives in the A & E department with her stepfather at 6.00 p.m. The history given by the stepfather is that Julie fell over the doorstep and hit her face on the chair in the kitchen. Julie has tears in her eyes (she is holding on to the stepfather), a swollen nose and blood around her mouth. She is taken to an examination cubicle.

Patient 7

David is 19 years of age. He arrives at 11.00 p.m. in the A & E department with several pals. All have been drinking heavily. A fight broke out in the pub and David has a small cut to his finger. The department is very busy but David and co. demand immediate attention and start to shout and disrupt the waiting-room.

Patient 8

Mr Cook is 50 years of age. He arrives by ambulance. Mr Cook is drowsy complaining of severe pain in his chest. He describes the pain as crushing and radiating to his neck and arms. Skin colour is pale, cold and clammy. Respiration is 22. Pulse is 80. Blood pressure is 100/60. The cardiac monitor shows sinus rhythm with ventricular ectopics. Mr Cook is complaining of nausea.

What assessment would you make regarding the history and appearance of Julie?

How do you deal with David and his pals?

Mr Cook suddenly collapses and appears not to be breathing, what do you do?

Julie, Patient 6

The first major observation is that although tears are in the eyes, Julie is not actively crying. There appears to be a bond between Julie and the stepfather.

In the examination room the nurse would first gain Julie's confidence by talking to her, using a toy as a tool to create the partnership. The nurse should ask Julie how she fell and consider her explanation in relationship with the injury. The nurse should ask if Julie could see clearly and if she could follow her finger with her eyes. The nose would be assessed for any bleeding and the mouth would be inspected. The nurse would check to see if the frenulum had been damaged.

Julie would be undressed. The nurse would support this action by explaining to the stepfather that children can often injure themselves elsewhere, while falling and not be aware of the injury. The stepfather's reaction would be noted. Is he concerned about the examination?

A careful examination of Julie's body would be made. Any bruises. Bite marks. Finger marks or hand prints should be considered.

POINTS TO CONSIDER

1 Why is the mother not with Julie?
2 Why is Julie not crying and cuddling the stepfather?
3 Is there a torn frenular?
4 Are there any marks on Julie's body?
5 Does the history fit the injury?

David, Patient 7

The most important move in this situation is to isolate David for his initial assessment. Communication is going to be difficult, but by being positive with David, this will help. Explain that you will assess his wound and medical care will be based on that and not the noise he or his pals make. Assess the wound.

There is very mild pain. The wound was caused by a piece of glass. The wound is a clean cut wound. There is no tissue loss and it is only superficial in depth. No foreign body could be seen and no tendon or other underlying structural damage appears to have occurred. During this assessment the partnership that had developed suggested that David and his pals were more high-spirited due to the alcohol than violent nature. This allows a more positive approach to be taken. David should be sent into the waiting-room having first had a temporary dressing applied to the wound. He should be told that while you will tolerate a few songs and general high spirits, if he or any of his pals become disruptive, the police will be called. As soon as possible David should be attended to by the doctor and discharged.

Mr Cook, Patient 8

The most important assessment is of the respiratory and circulatory system. Is respiratory arrest present? Is cardiac arrest present?

1 Patient is unconscious.
2 Patient is not breathing.

3 Patient is pale/cyanosed.
4 No carotid or femoral pulse is felt.

Monitor rhythm shows ventricular fibrillation.

INTERVENTION

Immediately summon help. Lie the patient flat. If authorized, defibrillate the patient 200 J ensuring all safety precautions are taken.

If not authorized to defibrillate or if defibrillation is unsuccessful, commence external ventilation and cardiac massage. Give a hard sternal thump. Give two slow deep ventilations. Check carotid pulse. If absent commence external chest compression, 15 compressions. As soon as a colleague is in attendance, work at a ratio of one ventilation to five chest compressions. Defibrillate as per departmental policy.

Conclusion

For too long, accident and emergency nurses have debated which model of nursing is appropriate for use in the department, what type of documentation to use, and how to develop accident and emergency as a true specialty. I hope through this book to have given some answers to these major issues and helped clear the way for the development of a specific process of accident and emergency care in every department in the UK.

The last three chapters have shown how the model of nursing combined with a triage system and a problem-orientated approach can provide a more logical and structured system of care, while at the same time allowing a sound basis for educating staff of all grades and experience.

I would encourage all readers to analyse the current systems of care in their department and where necessary make the appropriate changes before others with little or no accident and emergency nursing experience change your department for you.

References and further reading

AGGLETON P., CHALMER H., 'Models and Theories', *Nursing Times*, 5 September 1984–3 April 1985.

BALY M., *Nursing & Social Change*, Heinemann, London, 1973.

BLYTHIN P., 'Triage in the UK', *Nursing*, 1988; 3, 16.

BLYTHIN P., 'Triage: a nursing care system' in *Management and Practice in Emergency Nursing* (ed. Wright, B.), Chapman and Hall, London, 1988.

CARNEVALI, D., *Concepts Basic to Nursing*, McGraw-Hill, New York, 1973.

DANIS D., 'Professional development of nursing practice', in *Management and Practice in Emergency Nursing* (ed. Wright, B.), Chapman and Hall, London, 1988.

ELLIS M., *The Casualty Officer's Hand Book*, Butterworths, London, 1975.

FARROW R., *The Nursing of Accidents*, Unibooks, 1964.

HAZZARD, M. E. and KERGIN, D. J., 'Overview of system theory', *Nursing Choices of North America*, 6, 3, 1971.

HUNT S., 'Old Style Casualties, Survival Against the Odds', *Emergency Nurse*, V. 1985; 1.

JANIS, I., *Stress and Frustration*, Harcourt Brace, New York, 1971.

JOHNSON, D., (1975) Cited in Reehl, J. and Roy, C., *Conceptual Models for Nursing Practice*, Chapter 1, Appleton Century Crofts, New York, 1975.

JONES G., 'Top priority', *Nursing Standard*, 1988; 3, 28.

JONES G., 'Behind the Times', *Nursing Times*, 1986; 15 October, 30.

JONES G., *Learning to Care in the A & E Department*, Hodder and Stoughton, Sevenoaks, 1986.

McGUINNESS S., 'Sudden death in the emergency department', in *Management and Practice in Emergency Nursing* (ed. Wright, B.), Chapman and Hall, London, 1988.

NIGHTINGALE F., *Notes on Nursing*, Dover, 1969.

PEARSON A., VAUGHAN, B., *Nursing Models for Practice*, Heinemann, London, 1986.

RAMBO B., *Adaptation Nursing*, Saunders, New York, 1984.

Royal College of Surgeons of England, *Report of the Working Party on the Management of Patients with Major Injuries*, Royal College of Surgeons, London, 1988.

RUND D., RAUSCH T., *Triage*, Moseby, 1981.

RUTHERFORD, W., *Journal British Association of Immediate Care*, 12, 3, 1989.

SUCHMANN, Cited in Butterworth, C. A., *The Nursing Process – An Introduction and Overview* (unpublished observations), 1976.

WALSH M., *Accident and Emergency Nursing, A New Approach*, Heinemann, London 1985.

WRIGHT B., *Caring in Crisis*, Churchill Livingstone, London, 1986.

WRIGHT B., 'Encountering hostility and aggression' in *Management and Practice in Emergency Nursing* (ed. Wright, B.), Chapman and Hall, London, 1988.

WRIGHT S., *Building and Using a Model of Nursing*, Edward Arnold, 1986.

Working Documents/Published Guidelines

Nursing Care Plans for Patients in Emergency Department, a Working Document Published by The Registered Nurses Association of British Columbia.

Nursing Process and Triage in the Accident & Emergency Department, published by the Accident & Emergency Nursing Forum of the Royal College of Nursing.

Unpublished Work

COOK I., *Individualised Care/Basildon & Thurrock's Model of Nursing*, 1988.

GREEN L., *A Study of Nursing Care of an Elderly Patient Following a Colles's Fracture Using Orem's Model of Care*, Diploma in Nursing Work. Unit 6, 1989.

JONES G., *Accident Emergency Nursing in Canada and the USA*. (Available through the National Florence Nightingale Committee of GB and NI), 1980.

Index